BALINT MATTERS

BALINT MATTERS
Psychosomatics and the
Art of Assessment

Jonathan Sklar

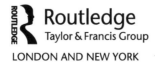

Routledge
Taylor & Francis Group

LONDON AND NEW YORK

First published 2017 by
Karnac Books Ltd.

Published 2018 by Routledge
2 Park Square, Milton Park, Abingdon, Oxon OX14 4RN
711 Third Avenue, New York, NY 10017, USA

Routledge is an imprint of the Taylor & Francis Group, an informa business

British Library Cataloguing in Publication Data

A C.I.P. for this book is available from the British Library

ISBN-13: 9781782204862 (pbk)

Typeset by V Publishing Solutions Pvt Ltd., Chennai, India

To E. B.

CONTENTS

PART II: BALINT GROUPS

PART III: ASSESSMENT

PATIENTS WHO APPEAR MORE THAN ONCE

Miss A

Mr C

Mrs E

ACKNOWLEDGMENTS

I want to thank all the doctors, general practitioners, psychiatrists, and paediatricians who have presented their clinical work and discussed their thoughts, feelings, and free associations about the clinical work with me in the contexts of working in Balint groups. And, of course, their patients, without whose contributions the enterprise would always fail.

As well as my dear friends Christopher Bollas and Michael Parsons, who always have had important perspectives on matters clinical and theoretical, I want to thank my colleagues who have listened to and critiqued various of these writings in my London Continuous Professional Development (CPD) group: Roger Kennedy, Rosemary Davies, Elizabeth Wolf, and Josh Cohen, as well as colleagues in the 1952 Club. Examining assessments has allowed particularly vigorous discussion in my Zurich CPD group, comprising of Peter Wegner, Eva Schmid-Gloor, and Denny Panitz. I have been in clinical and theoretical discussions in the Chicago groups that I have been convening now for many years, and to all those colleagues I am very grateful for their giving me the opportunity to discover the inflections of a North American understanding. Similarly, my thanks go to Mark and Karen Solms and my many South African colleagues for their inspirations annually over the last decade and more. Lene Auestad, having read many of the chapters, was able to offer a wider sociological and philosophic direction. Helen Johnson read the manuscript and helpfully commented. Thanks also to Ian Bostridge for his translation of *Der Leiermann in Winterreisse*. Jacqueline Rose read many of the chapters and her perceptive comments and discussions were very valuable to the project.

I am particularly grateful to Patrick Davies for his excellent realisations about what I meant to write, and his scholarship. Oliver Rathbone and Karnac have been patient with the long time coming of this manuscript.

Excerpt from Heaney, S. (1996). "Mycenae Lookout". In: *The Spirit Level*. London: Faber & Faber. Reprinted with kind permission of Faber & Faber.

Excerpt from Eliot, T. S. (1936). "Burnt Norton". In: *Collected Poems 1909–1935*. London: Faber & Faber, 1969. Reprinted with kind permission of Faber & Faber.

Excerpt from Müller, W. (1824). "The Hurdy-Gurdy Man". In: I. Bostridge (Trans.), *Schubert's Winter Journey: Anatomy of an Obsession*. London: Faber & Faber, 2015. Reprinted with kind permission of the translator.

Excerpt from Cavafy, C. P. (1928). In a large Greek colony, 200 BC. In: G. Savidis (Ed.), *Collected Poems*. London: Chatto & Windus, 1990. Reprinted with kind permission of Penguin Books Ltd.

Excerpt from Camus, A. (1942). *The Myth of Sisyphus*. London: Hamish Hamilton, 1955. Reprinted with kind permission of Penguin Books Ltd.

Excerpt from Berger, J. (1967). *A Fortunate Man: The Story of a Country Doctor*. London: Allen Lane [reprinted London: Canongate, 2015]. Copyright John Berger and Jean Mohr, 1967. Reprinted with kind permission of Canongate Books Ltd.

Excerpt from Mandela, N. (1964). Brief notes in the event of a death sentence. In: A. Sampson, *Mandela: The Authorised Biography*. London: Harper Collins, 1999. Reprinted with kind permission of the Nelson Mandela Foundation.

The epigraph by Thomas Ogden is taken from *The Primitive Edge of Experience* by Thomas Ogden (published by Karnac Books in 1992), and is reprinted with kind permission of Karnac Books.

The Chapter "Regression and new beginnings: Michael, Alice, and Enid Balint, and the circulation of ideas" was originally published in 2012 in the *International Journal of Psycho-analysis*, 93: 1017–1034. Copyright Institute of Psychoanalysis, 2012. This has now been reworked and is included with the kind permission of John Wiley and Sons Ltd.

ABOUT THE AUTHOR

Jonathan Sklar, MBBS FRCPsych, is a training analyst and fellow of the British Psychoanalytical Society. Originally trained in psychiatry at Friern and the Royal Free Hospitals, he trained for four years in adult psychotherapy at the Tavistock Clinic in London. For many years he was consultant psychotherapist and head of the psychotherapy department at Addenbrooke's and Fulbourn hospital in Cambridge. He now works in full-time analytic practice in London. He teaches and supervises at the Institute of Psychoanalysis; taught an MSc course for many years on "Ferenczi and Contemporary Psychoanalysis" at University College London; and teaches regularly in Chicago. For the past ten years he and Mark Solms have convened a psychoanalytic conference outside Cape Town and, for thirty years, he has convened Balint groups working with general practitioners and psychiatrists. He has lectured widely throughout East and West Europe and North America. His psychoanalytic papers have been published in Italian, Spanish, French, and Portuguese. From 2007 to 2011 he was Vice President of the European Psychoanalytic Federation. He was elected to the board of the International Psychoanalytical Association in 2015.

INTRODUCTION

During the past twenty-five years the Hungarian psychoanalyst Michael Balint has become something of a lost figure. This book endeavours to revive interest in his thinking and to re-establish his ideas that emphasised the value of making connections between psychoanalytic thinking, family medicine, and psychosomatics. Fragments of his ideas, such as "new beginnings", the "basic fault", and "Balint groups", are still known today, but often without the understanding of their original meaning and context. Through examining his radical ideas, I argue that they are of particular significance to us today, in our world of quick fixes and the overspecialisation of medicine. On coming to London, to the Tavistock Clinic, and the British Psychoanalytical Society, Balint continued the development of the ideas of his master, Sándor Ferenczi, and of the Budapest School of Psychoanalysis, building on and making key contributions to the theory and practice of the Independent tradition. In my earlier book, *Landscapes of the Dark* (2011), I examined the contributions of both Ferenczi and Balint to the field of regression and to our understanding of the process of being with patients suffering from severe, early traumatic states of mind. Here, I will examine Balint's exploration of what psychoanalysis and psychoanalytic thinking can contribute to general medicine, giving particular consideration to the impact of his theories on family practice.

Medicine today is becoming increasingly specialised. One manifestation of this trend is the widening gap between theories of the psyche and theories of the somatic. The idea and possibility of practising whole-person medicine is now regarded as rather old-fashioned. The Victorian idea of asylum for patients who need to be away from their lives for a period of time, in order to return after some restoration, is a similarly outmoded idea. For the twenty-first century, pharmaceutical medication is a much easier notion, allowing the omission of the importance of states of mind and feelings. The era of the internet has led us to expect knowledge to arrive instantly, and this has become confused with intelligence and thoughtfulness, as if the antiquated process of taking time to think only delays implementation, disrupting process and solution.

In an analogous manner, the arrival of Sigmund Freud's theories of the unconscious in the late nineteenth century was met with enormous professional disdain. Physicians and psychiatrists disagreed with the notion of a level of unconscious thought lying beneath a well-developed rationality. Night dreams, day dreams, neurotic symptoms, sexuality, perverse thoughts, and somatisation could, in the Freudian system of the unconscious, find a locus that made connections to previously separate matters. Perhaps the idea of so many diverse things—some clearly medical or psychiatric, and others regarded as peculiar, esoteric, or even irrelevant—being able to come into focus and achieve coherence has been part of the problem of the acceptance, then and now, of the force of psychoanalytic thinking. Building on the theory of the unconscious, if one links a patient's early history and the development of their mind with expectations of the specific patterns of those early relationships, a complex model can be assembled. If this is then discussed, a new sense can emerge of being understood by the analyst. Or, further, the patient may have the sensation that these ideas are not really new, but have a resonance that Christopher Bollas succinctly described as becoming aware of an unthought known. When the patient begins to notice connections between their symptoms and the history of their inner self and character, this process ignites a feeling of curiosity. The clinical atmosphere of listening, and of connecting disparate unconscious associations, can leave the patient feeling emotionally "held"—the process of beginning to be understood. The antipathy to such clinical directions can be enormous, however, as if such an articulation is too emotionally expensive to even contemplate.

Psychiatric wards have been subject to widespread closures, replaced with the slogan of "community care"—as if the patient is truly cared for within the community. Tablets are regarded as a more effective option, often prescribed and swallowed for many years. Contact between patient and doctor is certainly diminished. The now-global pharmaceutical industry commands vast resources, and can market their products more in pursuit of their own profits than to maintain high standards of healthcare. Psychiatric drug treatments are recommended for continuous prescription over many years. Often, the general practitioner is expected to continue the drug regime suggested by the psychiatrist, with the anxiety that if the treatment is stopped the patient will return to their former state, or even become worse. The whole underpinning of the *Diagnostic and Statistical Manual of Mental Disorders* (American Psychiatric Association, 2013) is corrupted by a pharmaceutical industry that creates new illnesses so that they can sell new drugs. Blushing, shyness, anger, sadness, and particularly mourning, amongst many other human characteristics, are now targeted states of mind that seem to require medication. Surrounding this trend is an atmosphere that such care does not require much in the way of resources. The severe paring down of psychiatric finances, from the budget of the NHS, seems to have at its core the diminution of the idea that the patient needs a place to think, express emotion, and be. Today, few resources exist for this enlightened, Victorian approach. Psychologists are expected to practise some sort of psychological therapy, although most will not have much specific training in dialogues with the patient. Counsellors now only generally offer about five or six sessions to deal with complex difficulties. In addition, their training for treating very ill patients is relatively brief. This is just another cheap resource that relies on, and even demands, the brevity of any therapeutic dyad. In this scenario the psychiatrist has rather little to contribute, especially once they have prescribed a regime of medication. This, in turn, has led to an internal dilemma for the psychiatrist that feels their role rapidly dissipating—listening to the patient being regarded as less important, readily deferred onto the nurse, psychologist, or counsellor. Usually, the patient is promptly returned to their general practitioner.

In today's practice, though, with more expectation and demand from both hospital and society, what can the general practitioner do with the patient that is returned still unwell? Michael Balint proposed a solution of listening to the patient in the holistic form of both mind and body, grounded in a psychoanalytic understanding. This did not mean reproducing the role of the psychoanalyst, seeing the patient for a fifty-minute session every day. Rather, Balint sought ways of listening to the ordinary discourse of a standard ten-minute consultation and, more particularly, realised that the doctor's own thoughts and feelings have a resonance that can be usefully employed to understand the patient. In analytic theory this is described as countertransference. Balint is the founding father of this whole-person general practice that gathers connections between the patient's immediate ailment, their early life and difficulties, their somatic illness, and their present state of mind. By bringing together general practice and psychoanalysis, Balint brought the general practitioner to the centre of the clinical debate—most manifestly in the form of Balint groups, in which general practitioners discussed the problems that they had with their patients. This was Balint's radical realignment of the "clinical problem" that the patient brought to the doctor. From the 1950s through to the 1990s the doctor really did function as the family practitioner, with knowledge of the dynamics of particular families' lives, from pregnancy to death, and from grandchildren to grandparents. This vast web of the complexity and emotional colouration of a family's life was known well by the doctor, a familiarity tacitly accumulated over many years. As a participant in the intimacies of the family, the doctor was a trusted receptacle for such knowledge, respected as having a privileged role in the family. It was this long-developed knowledge of a family that Balint was intent on activating— a vital part of the family that could be known outside of the family itself, allowed to gather in the unconscious mind of the doctor. The practice of the Balint group enabled that body of unconscious knowledge of the patient and their family to manifest itself more intensively in the crisis experienced by a doctor faced with a muddled and complicated case. The result was not to refer the patient on to the usual expert, such as a psychiatrist, or to prescribe their types of medication, but to encourage the doctor to face his or her own thoughts about the case—thoughts that could be beyond the realm of orthodox clinical practice. This was the influence of psychoanalytic thinking, provoking the utilisation of a doctor's deep connection with the life of his or her patient so that the doctor in themselves became the medicine, through the clinical interaction. In addition, the family doctor was allowed to touch the body of the patient in the expectation of a physical examination, which was impossible for the practising psychoanalyst. Here was another important strand that could be thought about in terms of the psychosomatic: the doctor physically placing hands on the patient contrasted with the analytic holding environment, an imaginary space of enabling the analysand to be "held". For Balint, general practice was a distillation of intimacy and knowledge with unconscious components in phantasy and somatisation, also enabling the doctor to be unconsciously perceived in a transference role, usually, although not necessarily, of a parent. All in all, Balint's suggestions posit a heady mix of depth and substance that could make the family doctor a powerful tool with extensive healing capabilities. With general medicine and psychoanalysis in dialogue, the doctor might take clinical control of complex psychiatric and psychosomatic cases. This could achieve much more than the current trend of referral to outside services that lack the depth of knowledge the general practitioner can have of his or her patients.

In our modern world, however, the family doctor is becoming something of a mythic character. The next doctor with a vacancy will see the next waiting patient. At a stroke, the deep, intimate history of a long-observed family life are eliminated from the clinical encounter. Symptoms are related to the next doctor that the patient sees, invariably as isolated phenomena, and certainly disconnected from emotional or family life. Perhaps one can argue the issue by suggesting that heart pain, or the onset of diabetes, or the difficulty of becoming pregnant are just physiological or genetic matters that do not need to be connected to the wider life of the patient, but patients still value being emotionally understood by their doctor, at the very least. Often taking such a singular path will be effective enough. But, for many patients, particularly the appropriately named "heart-sink" patients—complex and seemingly irresolvable cases which the doctor feels are stuck—the complexity of psychoneurotic and psychosomatic states of mind can be more appropriately understood and treated with a variant of the talking cure. In addition, the talking cure gives the doctor confidence in their clinical practice and allows them to rightly feel that their clinical skills include listening and speaking in a mode usually thought to exist only in the realm of the analyst. The onset of heart pain is significantly connected with difficulties in emotional life—"intimacies of the heart", as Marcel Proust would describe in relation to the problems of memory (Proust, 1921, p. 153). Indeed, at the onset of many physical illnesses it is always worth considering wider influences in the life of the patient that may have preceded the onset of symptoms. Arguably, the lowering of one's immune state that can allow a virus or bacteria to flourish may be connected to the patient's state of mind—a particular anxiety or depressive condition that implicitly and silently impacts on the efficacy of the immune system. The direct contact that the general practitioner and patient both expect to continue right through the generational family, from grandparents down to grandchildren, through all the specific vicissitudes in life—and even the ways the particular family deals with birth, separations, and death—is something the doctor collects over many years, taking an interest in the family for decades. It takes just a second to conjure up that knowledge as the known patient enters their consulting room, or at the beginning of a home visit. Yet, this instant recall of the family in the mind of their doctor is currently being destroyed, as if it has no relevance in modern clinical medicine. It is the medical equivalent of the analyst's imaginative holding of the patient.

This book falls into three parts. The first two provide a history of Michael and Enid Balint's contributions to medicine, with Part I giving an introduction to their theoretical perspective, and Part II describing the Balint group's methodology, and providing many clinical vignettes from groups I have convened with general practitioners. Balint's history and his wide impact across the field of psychoanalysis stems from his beginnings in Budapest and his analysis with Ferenczi, as well as the bringing of his master's papers and clinical diary when he fled to London in 1938—thus preserving and keeping alive the important Hungarian contribution to psychoanalysis, with Ferenczi's specific developments and particular interest in early states of mind, trauma, and the analysis of the child in the adult. He began this work by listening to general practitioners in Budapest, and in the early 1950s set up such groups at the Tavistock Clinic in London. He was soon joined by his wife, Enid and together they developed the methodology of Balint groups. In 1983, I applied this method to the training of junior psychiatrists for the first time. This book includes another series of short case studies that serve to illustrate how the young psychiatrist can begin to understand the psychodynamics of his or her patient through the prism of their own specific difficulty with the case as a doctor. In a similar vein, I offer an example of a Balint group in South Africa, attended by obstetricians and paediatricians, that found itself entangled in the awful dilemmas of HIV. This chapter highlights both the broad applicability of Balint's methodology and the depth of its impact on participants—in this case helping them to think amidst the severe pressures of a society in the grip of post-apartheid and the AIDS epidemic, and in a social reality that encouraged projection onto the doctor. In this section I also document Balint's profound interest in the training of psychoanalysts, which was, he recognised, an indispensable point of discussion when considering the future of psychoanalysis. I have therefore included a chapter discussing some contemporary perspectives on the inherent difficulties involved in the pursuit of an analytic training.

The third part of the book addresses the importance of the initial psychodynamic assessment. I describe the complex processes involved in assessment and attempt to offer a "road map" with which to delineate the different aspects of the work. In doing so, I examine the territory of this form of assessment in great detail, taking the first few minutes of the interaction as a crucial template for how to begin the process itself. An early memory from the patient can provide an invaluable etching of resonances from early life, and from the development of object relationships. Other elements include focusing on a particular dream, and also examining the sexual life of the patient, considering its impact on the history of the individual's character and on their capacity for intimacy, along with possible connections to psychopathology. All this falls within the envelope of Balint's interest in understanding the early childhood and adolescence of the patient, and the essential value of such history in beginning to make sense of the psychosomatic symptoms and anxieties that the patient suffers from. Finally, this section describes the termination of the assessment process and what to do with the found synthesis when deciding the appropriate form of treatment. In all of these chapters, I provide an abundance of clinical vignettes to aid understanding of the theoretical structures. Some examples are referred to throughout in an attempt to provide a sense of continuity, particularly in terms of assessment as conducted through the different phases of the clinical procedure. The value of this descriptive journey through the process of assessment does not reside solely in its relevance for analysts in training, who often find themselves introduced to this skill at quite a late stage of their clinical education. If knowledge of this process is of value to analytic psychotherapists, it may also be useful to the psychiatrist, general practitioner, psychologist, and social worker. Here, we return full circle to Balint, who was a profound and outspoken commentator on the pleasures and perils of psychoanalytic training, as well as on its wider social purpose outside the psychoanalytic consulting room. I believe that such forms of attention, by re-examining this wider purpose, can help open up a black box, superficially perceived with an increasingly prevalent assumption that these are arcane ideas reserved for the privileged use of psychoanalysts.

My reflections here are directed against the lightness of assessment increasingly familiar in today's psychiatric practice, reliant on genetic and behavioural underpinnings of psychopathology that do not require complex examination. This narrow focus has a circular effect, for if something is not searched for it will not be found, thus facilitating a justification against complex forms of patient assessment on the grounds that it appears to have no value. This is psychiatry (and, I would add, some general medical practice) at its most nihilistic and blind. At the same time, it is true that psychodynamic assessment is a difficult and sensitive operation, understandably becoming less popular due to its being inadequately taught. This in itself can provoke the fear that such investigation may further agitate the patient, perhaps worsening their particular state of mind. Such fears, however, are incongruent with the time-honoured medical lineage to which they often appeal—one which has always regarded the physical assessment of the patient to be an essential clinical tool, perhaps hurting the patient temporarily whilst palpating a sore and painful area but, in doing so, making diagnosis possible. Ideally, the exploration presented here will allow practitioners inside and outside of psychoanalysis to feel that they have an assessment map for the difficult task both of understanding what is happening in the clinical encounter and of trying to process so many obtuse strands. My hope, therefore, is that such an excursion into the labyrinth of psychodynamic assessment will be valuable, not only to therapists and psychiatrists but also, in the tradition of Michael Balint, to general practitioners and counsellors who wish to understand more of the realm of our unconscious.

PART I

AN OVERVIEW OF MICHAEL BALINT'S WORK

CHAPTER ONE

Regression and new beginnings: Michael, Alice, and Enid Balint, and the circulation of ideas

Who is crazy, we or the patients? (the children or the adults?)

—Sándor Ferenczi, *The Clinical Diary* (1932, p. 92)

Michael Balint was born Bergmann Mihály in Hungary on 3 December 1896 to a general-practitioner father. In 1920, he changed his name to Michael Balint, against his father's will, and converted to the Unitarian Religion, thus avoiding some sanctions imposed on Jews. Whilst studying medicine during the First World War he was called up for army service, during which he received a severe injury to his thumb that led to a claw-like deformity. In 1917 he was given Freud's *Totem and Taboo* by a young colleague, Alice Szekely-Kovacs, who had been a university classmate, together with Margaret Mahler (all would later become analytic colleagues). In 1918, Ferenczi was appointed to the first Chair of Psychoanalysis, and the young Balint attended the inaugural lecture series in 1919, just before the overthrow of Bela Kuhn's Communist Republic. Michael and Alice, now married a year later in 1920, fled the counter-revolution to Berlin, where Michael worked in the biochemical laboratory of Otto Warburg. By 1922 the couple had both started analytic training with Hanns Sachs in Berlin.

3

Balint regarded Sachs as too didactic an analyst—one who would nevertheless interrupt sessions by answering the phone (Stewart, 1996, p. 2). Two years later they then returned to Budapest, both commencing an analysis with Ferenczi, remaining with him for a further two years until he left Hungary for an eight-month lecture tour of the US. It was in Ferenczi's waiting room that Balint first came into contact with Melanie Klein. From 1925 he began publishing papers on psychoanalysis and assumed a leading role within the Hungarian psychoanalytic movement. By 1935, two years after Ferenczi's death, Balint became director of the Budapest Psychoanalytic Institute. Following the Anschluss of Austria in 1938, he and Alice made arrangements to flee to Britain with their son. They were aided by Ernest Jones, who in 1939 helped them to settle, not in London as desired, but in Manchester. Within a few months of their arrival, however, Alice suddenly died of a ruptured aneurysm—a condition under whose shadow they had lived for several years. In 1945, Balint's parents, who had remained in Hungary, committed suicide to avoid being arrested by the Nazis. That year, Balint made the decision to move to London, where he obtained a Master of Science in psychology with a thesis entitled "Individual Differences in Early Infancy". If we consider this brief early history from a Ferenczian perspective, one is able to trace elements of Balint's traumatic landscape: a hand deformed by war, forsaking his father's name, twice escaping from home and country, and the sudden death of his wife and both parents within a few short years. Such traumata involving the self, the other, and the environment would become profound topics of debate in his subsequent writings, which were developed amidst the growing influence of notions of early object relationships.

Alongside this personal and geographic history, it is useful to give an initial summary of Balint's prominent relationship with the tradition of psychoanalysis that preceded him. Balint became Ferenczi's literary executor, and when travelling to England brought with him, amongst many documents and papers, the original manuscript of *The Clinical Diary*, which covered the last year of Ferenczi's life and his private thoughts on the clinical and theoretical gap that had opened up between him and Freud from late 1932. Balint transcribed and translated this valuable record into English. He also had possession of Freud's letters to Ferenczi, a collection forming half of that extraordinary correspondence. Devoting considerable effort to keeping the flame of Hungarian psychoanalytic thought alive, Balint strongly desired to publish the correspondence along with *The Clinical Diary*. Together they contained the core of the Budapest Psychoanalytical School and its historical development in association with Freud. Due to consideration for those individuals still living, however, including Anna Freud—who refused the publication of her father's half of the correspondence—Balint was unable to publish them in his lifetime. To touch on one central topic of this crucial set of correspondence, Freud had, in his later career, become cautious about the therapeutic efficacy of psychoanalysis (Ferenczi, 1932, p. 93). In contrast, Ferenczi was well-known for his enthusiasm for clinical work. Balint was to continue Ferenczi's research into themes such as the analytic setting, character analysis, and, in particular, the role of the analyst in the analytic environment, culminating in his final and most important book on regression, *The Basic Fault: Therapeutic Aspects of Regression* (1968). The other major strand of Balint's corpus—relating to his and Ferenczi's trust in clinical work—was the application of psychoanalytic thinking to the study of doctors and their interaction with patients. This resulted in his book *The Doctor, his Patient and the Illness* (1957), which he described in the introduction as "research-cum-training" (p. 3), and which became well-known amongst medical practitioners. What I am seeking to offer in this opening chapter is not merely an account of Balint's trajectory, but an examination of a moment in the history of the conceptualisation of psychoanalytic training and technique—and the controversies that have subsequently arisen.

The analytic pair

In terms of the understanding of psychoanalytic technique, one of Balint's particular contributions was to examine the process and the role of the analyst in establishing the character, range, and depth of the project of the analytic pair. As Jacques Lacan noted, Balint focused on understanding the fundamental object-relation, which he calls "primary love, namely the relations between mother and infant" (Lacan, 1975, p. 209). For Lacan, a key element in this understanding was provided by Alice Balint's paper "Love for the Mother and Mother Love" (1939), in which, theoretically, the mother satisfies all the needs of the infant. This complex scenario of real and imagined experience is the structural crucible on which all that follows is based. Alice Balint heroically demonstrates "that maternal need displays exactly the same limits as every vital need, namely that *when one no longer has anything to give, well one takes … *[I]n any given so-called primitive society … when there is nothing left to eat, you eat your child" (Lacan, 1975, p. 210, italics in original). His reading pays tribute to Alice Balint for recognising the negative component of this relation. Using this model as his template, while remaining perhaps more conventionally within its terms, Michael Balint based his account of primary love on the mother–infant relationship, in which the maternal object corresponds to the satisfaction of a need.

Masud Khan's shrewdly if cacophonously entitled essay "On the Clinical Provision of Frustrations, Recognitions, and Failures in the Analytic Situation: An Essay on Dr. Michael Balint's Researches on the Theory of Psychoanalytic Technique" (1969) draws a connection with Ferenczi's last controversial paper, "Confusion of Tongues Between Adults and the Child" (1933), and makes clear that Balint is the true heir of that Budapest strand of technique and theory. Central to Balint's conceptualisation is the idea of the "basic fault", a term used to describe the relatively common experience in early two-person relationships that something is wrong or missing, and that this has been carried over into the oedipal period (from two to five years old). In Balint's theory, resolution of the "basic fault" takes place through regression within the analytic setting. This is a subject that divides the analytic world today, with many colleagues regarding regression as antithetical or even dangerous to an analysis. For Balint, however:

> The analyst must accept the regression. This means that he must create an environment, a climate, in which he and his patient can tolerate the regression as a mutual experience … What the analyst must provide—and, if at all possible, during the regular sessions only—is sufficient time free from extrinsic temptations, stimuli, and demands, including those originating from himself (the analyst). The aim is that the patient should be able to find himself, to accept himself, and to get on with himself, knowing all the time that there is a scar in himself, his basic fault, which cannot be "analysed" out of existence; moreover, he must be allowed to discover his way to the world of objects—and not be shown the "right" way by some profound or correct interpretation … To provide this sort of object or environment is certainly an important part of the therapeutic task. Clearly, it is only a part, not the whole of the task. Apart from being a "need-recognizing" and perhaps even a "need-satisfying" object, the analyst must be also a "need-understanding" object,

who in addition must be able to communicate his understanding to his patient.

(M. Balint, 1968, pp. 177–181)

Balint is signalling a radical adaptation in technique in order to attempt to reach those patients who are unable to speak their distress in a language other than regression—an adaptation that will include enactment as well as psychosomatic defences as means of attempting to communicate beyond words. Rather than being fearful of the demands it might make on the analysis, and of not knowing where such a path may lead, Balint directs attention to the essential means of such communication as a furtherance, rather than a hindrance, to the analytic process.

New beginnings

To understand this, we need to go back to Balint's earliest ideas—specifically, to the concept of the "new beginning". He introduced this concept surprisingly early, at the 1932 Wiesbaden conference in which Ferenczi gave his last paper, the badly understood and poorly received "Confusion of the Tongues between Adults and the Child"—I have written much on Freud and Ferenczi's misunderstandings of each other's positions (Sklar, 2011, pp. 2, 40, & 69). From a historical perspective, Balint was already drawing attention to the clinical development of Ferenczi's analytical descriptions of the therapeutic dyad in arrested development. For some patients, in the childhood situation a complementary factor was that the child's trust had been betrayed. When the patient repeats this in analysis the analyst's passive unobtrusiveness alone can help the patient drop his self-protective character structure. For Balint, this constituted the experience of the "new beginning". Such patients, due to earlier loss or traumatic environments, give expression to the need for that which was felt to be missing—more particularly, a missing form of being. This missing state is the precondition for object-relating, meaning that achieving it will enable the patient to be in a condition to both offer and receive object-love, very often for the first time in their life.

For Ferenczi, particular levels of tension, described with a metaphor of elasticity, were sometimes essential for the development of the analytic process (Ferenczi, 1928, pp. 87–101). Freud agreed with the idea of elasticity as a description of the analyst's tact (ibid., p. 99). Evolving this theme, Balint continued to write about this necessary elasticity in technique (M. Balint, 1950, pp. 117–124). In relation to such flexibility and sensitivity, in his contribution to honour Melanie Klein on her seventieth birthday in an issue of the *International Journal of Psychoanalysis*, he described new beginnings that occur near the end of analysis as: "reactions which can be observed and recognized only with difficulty, as the level of pleasure amounts only to a *tranquil quiet sense of well-being*" (M. Balint, 1952, p. 215, italics in original). For more ill patients it is likely that such an atmosphere was rarely available in the early stages of their life, if at all. For Balint, analytic work can enable a new chapter of life and relationships to be available to the analysand, who, whilst fully cognisant of prior defences against early traumatic impingements, can nonetheless move away from the grip of these past fixities and expectations. In Balint's own summation,

> new beginning means the capacity for an unsuspicious, trusting, self-abandoned and relaxed object-relation. There are two clinically necessary conditions without which a proper phase of new beginning cannot develop. These are: (*a*) the relinquishing of the paranoid attitude, the realization that the paranoid anxieties were unfounded or at least grossly exaggerated; (*b*) the acceptance, without undue anxiety, of a certain amount of depression as an inevitable condition of life.
>
> (M. Balint, 1952, p. 220)

Here we find the roots of Balint's exposition of primary love as a form of love that is earlier than and free of the Kleinian death drive, postulated as early aggression, and envy by the baby of the breast. In relation to such negative early experience, Balint took issue with previous notions of developmental chronology, arguing that particular defensive structures are acquired in relation to early environmental impingements and traumas. For Klein, "the first phase of the human mind is dominated by paranoid anxieties and mechanisms and … this is followed by the depressive position" (M. Balint, 1952, p. 221). In this paper, Balint characterised these arguments about early development in a to-and-fro discourse that remains theoretically open rather being entrenched in politics—those of either a particular psychoanalytic theory or a particular analytic group. He does not idealise theory but sets out how complicated it can become. Whilst he praised Klein for her valuable contributions about working with children, he did not agree with her view of the death drive as an early given and as a bedrock of the mind. He believed that clinical techniques should evolve through the challenge of the patient's history and through the dynamics between archaic object-love and the early environment—dynamics to be exposed within the analytic process.

For Balint, in contrast to Klein, pathological narcissism was always secondary to trauma, and he disagreed with the formulation of early object relations as starting with the death drive, seeing this as an instinctual reductionism. Klein's destructive force, residing in each individual and tending towards the annihilation of life, was represented by greed, destructive envy, and omnipotent denial of dependence—all of which, for her school, coexist from uterine life. Balint thought that archaic object-love was only underdeveloped, such that the analytic task was to assist its growth. Remarking on complexity well beyond a Kleinian split of the object into just good and bad, he described "unsuspicious, naïve, archaic object-love" as "the first post-natal phase in the development of the human mind; it is a centre or nodal point from which all later developments radiate" (M. Balint, 1952, p. 223). One development from this primary stage would then be narcissism, as developing according to the environmental provision—meaning the amount of trauma that may have occurred, due, say, to the mother's impingements. Eventually, he argues, "the depressive position must be considered more fundamental, more primitive, than the paranoid" (ibid., p. 224).

A digression on the death instinct

Before ending this section, I would like to introduce Paula Heimann, who qualified as an analyst in Berlin in 1933 with a classical Freudian training, after which she immediately had to flee to London. There she soon became interested in Klein's work and underwent further training with her. In time, she became one of Klein's closest associates, and her early papers are clear expositions of Kleinian concepts: sublimation and creativity (1942), the internal object (1949), and the early stages of the oedipal complex (1952). But from around 1949 she began to move away from Klein, becoming critical of the theory of the death drive and of early aggression. Eventually, as outlined by Margret Tonnesman, Heimann

> viewed severe pathological states, like psychotic depressions, as regressions to early death-like somatic traumata with lack of differentiation of self and object and extreme cruelty operative in the patient's inner world. In her ... paper, "Notes on the anal stage", she suggested re-naming the anal-sadistic phase of development the anal-locomotor phase, as sadism and cruelty point to failure in the environmental facilitation during this phase of development.
>
> (Tonnesmann, 1989, p. 19)

In this paper, Heimann relates to both Donald Winnicott's and Balint's views of the environment as provision that either holds or fails to hold. In a later paper, she goes on to illuminate the difference between Freud's theories of the life and death instincts. The natural position of human beings is to generally wish to survive, and to go on living.

> What, then, is the death instinct? There are many situations in which our patients tell us and show us that they want to be dead. I believe that it is more correct to say that they want to be dead than to say that they want to die; indeed, analysis reveals that the wish in question concerns a state that is painless, while the fact of dying is usually strongly invested with phantasies of pain. Behind the wish to be dead what one really finds is the wish to be free of pain, whether physical, or psychical, such as shame, guilt, intolerable fears, anxiety, depression, confusion, despair, and so on, or we find phantasy wishes to be revenged upon or to kill an object with which the patient has unconsciously identified. A fairly typical revenge phantasy, which is often pre-conscious, consists of imagining one's parents in a state of terrible guilt, suffering from remorse, accusing each other over their child's grave: here an Oedipal wish is concealed behind the wish to be dead.
>
> (Heimann, 1969, p. 253)

Here, Heimann is developing an understanding of death, away from a fundamental wish to return to an inanimate state, as described by Freud. Rather, the idea of being inanimate is primarily an expression of negativism, indifference, contempt for pain, and lack of self-interest. These are states of mind of an opposite formation to that of a creative life, fragments of dissociative mind—as found in psychosis, severe manic-depressive states, and perversion—which can start as intrusions of bad parenting in early infancy. Heimann eventually states: "Personally, what I no longer find convincing is the relation between the hypothetical death instinct and the primary destructive drive" (ibid., p. 255). The importance of this later work lies in its descriptions of her giving up the seductive pull of inertia and primary destructiveness. Kleinians regard the latter as a central concept, and see an analysis without such introspective theoretical discussion as superficial. I would argue that such a position distances the Kleinian analyst by diminishing the historical findings of the various intrusions into the bodies and minds of babies, children, and adolescents, discovered through the transference, as well as being a radically different theory of primary love championed by Balint. For the Balints, these intrusions constitute the traumatic substrate that can be found in the centre of the environment that is analysis and, when understood, can be overcome by the patient that discovers the possibility of a new beginning.

The basic fault

In his final book, *The Basic Fault* (1968), Balint examines the above dynamics in the regressed patient and their analyst. Here the word "fault" is used in a geographic sense, as in a fault line that may connect or disjoin underlying tectonic plates. The term functions as a metaphor for splits in the ego and for their subsequent development, including that within analytical treatment.

Let us start by examining Balint's text from the perspective of his theory of primary love, which describes experiences of harmony between the individual and the world. Donald Winnicott would describe one such similar area of harmony as a "good enough" feed, after which a devouring infant and a devoured mother are mutually satisfied in the moment. Balint argues that within this experience of satisfaction both mother and infant are "in a state of complete harmony ... [T]he individual does not care and is not in a position to say where he ceases and the external world begins" (M. Balint, 1959, p. 67). The infant, he writes, is "surrounded, almost floats, in substances without exact boundaries; the substances and the individual mutually penetrate each other; that is, they live in a harmonious mix-up" (ibid., p. 67). He describes the activity of creation similarly, in which there may be no object present and the subject creates only out of themselves—not just referring to artistic creativity, but also to the difficulty of attaining insight, which necessarily requires the presence of another.

Aware that such states can only be transient, due to the reality principle, Balint then describes two ways that separateness from the primary object is discovered: first, through what he calls the creation of an "ocnophilic world", consisting of an unconscious phantasy structure based on the conviction that firm objects are reliable, kind, and available when needed; and, second, through an opposite unconscious phantasy that holds to the possibility of a "philobatic world" prior to the harmonious state, in which objects are experienced as dangerous, unpredictable, or to be got rid of (ibid., p. 68). However, if in early life the child senses that the object (mother) does not actually have real concern for the self, there is the possibility of a creative drive which emerges from the child's singularity as a person, and which is not an object relationship of care and love. This would be the position of the artist that creates a canvas as a means of surviving being alone, out of necessity, making their mark on the empty canvas as an expression of the notion that they are there—despite not being perceived by the (consistently preoccupied) maternal object. As well as such creative strategies there can also be pathological developments, such as psychosis, applied as an imaginative patch to the ego in order to cope with and manage being unperceived and unseen by the mother.

In relation to his strange Latinisms, Balint's therapeutic vision was that, in accepting regression, the patient was granted a right to free themselves from perceived oppressive objects in order to rediscover "the friendly expanses of the philobatic world demanding the possession of adult skills, and behind it the world of primary love which holds one safely without making any further demands on one" (ibid., p. 103). Whilst it is clear that the analyst may need to weather the storms of a paranoid transference, it is part of the expectation of the analyst that such necessary testing is essential for the analysand to realise that they are in the presence of a new object who, contrary to early experience, can be unexpectedly available for a quiet and unoppressive "feed". From now on the analysand's world does not have to function within the usual phantasy of dangerous objects perpetually encroaching on the self. The difficulties of achieving this state depend firmly on the capacity of the analyst to accept and bear the unfolding regressions.

If the analyst moves too quickly to reinstate an integrative state, the free-associative capacities within the enactments of the regression will be unavailable to contribute to new understanding. It might allow the analyst to be more comfortable, but what of the patient?

Balint described several ways that he saw as negatively curtailing clinical work to the level of the Oedipus complex, despite the patient's need to regress. One was for the analyst to pronounce the patient as unanalysable. Another, in debate with the Kleinians, was for the patient to conform to an analyst who has developed a certain style of knowing and a one-sided dynamic of telling the patient what is happening. Balint, in contrast, was interested in differentiating analytic work beyond and, indeed, prior to the level of the Oedipus complex. In the latter, the analysand is required to have a solid enough ego structure that contains early experiences of frustration: "interpretations are experienced by both patient and analyst as interpretations and not as something else" (M. Balint, 1968, p. 9). Such work is in the area of unconscious object-relating. However, for many patients, difficulties begin when they cannot bear or are suspicious of such a level of coherence or integration. Instead, it is more acceptable to be themselves by returning to what Balint described as a more primitive mental state. For Balint, this heralded a movement from the three-person oedipal level of functioning to a two-body psychology—one in which there is no capacity for triangulation, or even an ability to function with adult language.

This explicates one of Balint's key disagreements with Kleinian theory in regard to the paranoid-depressive position. For him, the handicap of this approach was that:

> Their interpretations—as reported at our scientific meetings and in the literature—create the impression of originating from a confident, knowledgeable, and perhaps even overwhelming analyst, an impression apparently shared by their patients. If true, this attitude of the analyst might be one of the reasons why, on the one hand, so much aggressiveness, envy, and hatred emerges in their patients' association-material and, on the other hand, why they seem to be concerned so much with introjection and idealization. These are the two most frequently used defence mechanisms in any partnership in which an oppressed, weak partner has to cope with an overwhelmingly powerful one.

(M. Balint, 1968, p. 107)

A third way that the analyst can curtail the regressive process valued by Balint would be to give in to an urge to over-organise the analysand's complaints into an illness (which, in itself, may contain a nidus of historical accuracy), rather than accepting a state of being with a patient who, for the present moment at least, can only exist in an unorganised mental state. For Balint, such disorganisation, which he aptly described as the "basic fault", should not be seen in terms of blame (of being "at fault"), but rather as a metaphor for a mental landscape. As I have previously written:

> In his 1924 paper *Neurosis and Psychosis*, Freud highlighted the delusion as a patch, thereby directing attention to the delusions, imaginary constructs, as well as fixities of the body ... that enable life apparently to continue on the surface as if there is no mental gap or tear. The symptoms are there as a covering structure to enable some sense of not fragmenting. The patch over the ego does not have a healing function, it is an unconscious phantasy because the deeper mental structures held apart from each other do not grow together. Instead, the patch can become more organized, such as a delusional system quietly enlarging to take account of the different unconscious narratives and relational affects on either side of the tear. Like dreams, this image of patchwork, if taken seriously, can become another royal road to understanding unconscious process through which the healing of deep splits, albeit with psychic scars, can occur.
>
> (Sklar, 2011, p. 9)

The clinical importance of such a stance is considerable. Instead of the patient experiencing constant disruption around the gap—whenever reality inevitably intrudes and as he vainly attempts to keep parts of the mind apart—the work with the unobtrusive analyst provides a new possibility of being with the other. It is not a question of whether the basic fault is a good thing or something to get rid of. Rather it is an early defensive state of being that, up until now, had protected the analysand, but with the price of maintaining a state of really being alone—despite a superficial view of living in a world populated with others. It is only by recognising the existence of this primitive state and allowing it to emerge on its own, usually disconnected with the other person, that, in time, the analyst can be perceived as being in the room. Then the analysand's move from being in a state of one-person psychology to being in a two-person relationship in the analysis becomes available, such that there is a possibility of regression.

Regression

The basic fault is characterised as possessing four features:

> (a) all the events that happen in it belong to an exclusively two-person relationship—there is no third person present; (b) this two-person relationship is of a particular nature, entirely different from the well-known human relationships of the Oedipal level; (c) the nature of the dynamic force operating at this level is not that of a conflict, and (d) adult language is often useless or misleading in describing events at this level.
>
> (M. Balint, 1968, pp. 16–17)

To add to this, states of deadness and emptiness can predominate (as we will see, this was a central insight of Enid Balint's work). The patient often has a conviction that something is the matter, that some wrong has been done, and that something requires redress. There is an atmosphere that the analyst must not let the patient down, and yet, paradoxically, is expected to do so. Sometimes, the analyst needs to work without doing anything other than just be. The patient may recognise that the analyst is still in the room by hearing their breathing, meaning that they are still alive and available to be made use of at some time. Any desire on the part of the analyst to clear tension with a knowledgeable interpretation is likely either to fail or to be falsely accepted. Knowing such a scenario of being with the patient and not needing to do anything more or do anything less may help the analyst be present in such a way that they seem not to be doing analytic work with the patient. Anything else done by the analyst at the level of the "basic fault" may be perceived by the patient as an attack, or deemed irrelevant. Balint concludes, "It is definitely a two-person relationship in which, however, only one of the partners matters; his wishes and needs are the only ones that count and must be attended to" (ibid., p. 23). This statement would also appear to make sense from the perspective that sometimes the patient is in a primitive defensive state of "one-person" psychology, as described by John Rickman: "'One-person psychology' concerns itself with what goes on inside one person taken in isolation" (Rickman, 1951, p. 218).

For Balint, hate and sadism are secondary factors in human development, taking the environmental provision seriously that they are consequences of inevitable frustration—increased in measure with early damage. The therapeutic process of regression involves both the analyst and the patient. The analyst cannot be only in the third position, viewing the conflict and interpreting it, since they themselves are part of it. Interpreting in the transference can only come as a later part of the work of analysis, when the patient has moved out of regression and is functioning at an oedipal level. As the state of regression is survived by the dyad, Balint describes the onset of an *arglos* (innocent) state. Here, the patient, now freer of both rigid and complex unconscious patterns and oppressive forms of relating, can begin to find a new way to relate to an object, as well as being capable of allowing an object to relate to themselves. The patient may then realise that they and the object are not reciprocally vulnerable to each other, and there can be a return to the state of primal love that preceded the detachment from the object world due to severe, early environmental failure.

It is important to note that Balint differentiates between benign and malignant regression. Malignant regression is aimed at gratification of instinctual cravings and is often to be understood as the patient seeking an external event or action in order to enhance, excite, or escape from their object. Gratification is the essential element here—the self's pleasure being of greater concern than any impact on the other. Balint differentiates this form of regression from a benign regression in which the patient expects to use the external world as a way of dealing with their internal difficulties—in Winnicott's terms, to be able to use the object. There can be difficulty in understanding Balint in this part of his work because there is a dearth of clearly differentiated clinical examples of the two types of regression. I am in agreement with Harold Stewart (1996, p. 74), who suggests that all the examples given are in the realm of the unobtrusive analyst with an analysand in a state of benign regression. Malignant regression is more uncooperative, greedy, violently envious, and destructive. In my reading of Enid Balint, I see her as regarding the movement from malignant to benign regression as being able to occur when the patient allows him or herself to feel alone, in the analyst's presence, but with an unconscious phantasy that no other person is present (E. Balint, 1989, p. 103). (She also usefully entwines Winnicott's discovery with Balint's work in regression.) The intense force of hatred directed towards the object in malignant regression can find no outlet for expression when the analyst does not exist for the patient but, paradoxically, is also present. It can take a long time before the patient unconsciously realises this state of absence/presence and, in time, they may dare to begin to trust the analyst enabling the transition from malignant regression to benign regression. During this time, the analyst must withstand both the patient's and their own hate. Probably particularly with his clinical collaboration with Enid, this process, as described by Winnicott (1947), was also known to Balint (1968, p. 71). Enid was very present in the writing of *The Basic Fault*, to which she brought her own ideas, including the experience of her analysis with Winnicott. My argument here is that the influence of that analysis, and of her earlier papers, especially her 1963 paper "On Being Empty of Oneself", from which Michael quotes (M. Balint, 1968, p. 19), can be seen in the shadows of her husband's famous book.

The area of creativity

The last part of Balint's theoretical development postulates an area of creativity in which there is no external object present and, therefore, which is without a transference relationship (M. Balint, 1968, p. 24). As this area is one that is non-verbal, Balint likened it to Bion's idea of beta function (ibid., p. 25). Coining the term "pre-object", Balint was interested in the task of enabling the pre-object to come into being as an object (ibid., p. 25). In Balint's words: "The last train of thought is connected with my ideas about the area of creation, an area of mind in which there is no external organized object, and any intrusion of such an object by attention-seeking interpretations inevitably destroys for the patient the possibility of creating something out of himself" (ibid., p. 176).

Balint describes the patient in such a state as appearing to be silent, withdrawn, seemingly "acting out", being repetitious, or regressing (ibid., p. 176). Whilst these observations might be valid, such behaviours may also be occurring whilst creative work is going on alone, separately from the analyst. Balint's point is that such states can be wrongly perceived as resistance, leading to a mistaken use of intervention that then fails the patient. The analyst can only "order" the material and offer interpretation after a return to the oedipal level. It is important that regression is first accepted and tolerated as a mutual experience. Lacan also accepted this understanding of presence in absence, but instead saw it as a linguistic phenomenon, critiquing the emphasis on the mother–infant dyad as neglectful of the symbolic function (Lacan, 1978). The point at question is Ferenczi's evocation of the child present in the adult, and how the former might be met and accepted in an analysis (Ferenczi, 1931). Clinically, the patient can move from being alone with their state of mind or illness to experiencing a new relationship in analysis, where notice of the external object's arrival allows an understanding to be expressed verbally—communication now able to occur in language, and taking place in work between the couple in the analytic setting.

Michael Balint died on 31 December 1970, whilst serving as President of the British Psychoanalytical Society. It is a major loss that he was unable to develop further many of the ideas described in his last book. I would suggest, however, that Michael Balint's theories on regression can be seen to be buttressed by Alice Balint's essential paper of 1939, "Love for the Mother and Mother Love", and also, half a century later, by Enid Balint's 1989 paper on "Creative Life", both of which add to a key dimension of his work.

Enid Balint's contribution

Enid Balint was first analysed by Rickman. He had himself been initially analysed by Freud in 1919; later, in 1928, by Ferenczi (Haynal, 2002, p. 127); and finally, in order to learn about Klein's theories when she had arrived in the British Psychoanalytical Society, with her too. Enid then had a second analysis with Winnicott and was in treatment until his death in 1971. The analytic theories active within her—including those of the Hungarian line, through Rickman, including his experiences in analysis with Freud and Klein—were refined and re-examined in her dialogues with Michael, whom she married in 1953.

I first want to discuss Enid Balint's paper "On Being Empty of Oneself" (1963a), which was published prior to *The Basic Fault*. Her thoughtfulness about misrecognition and its consequences—ideas that both she and Michael were certainly developing in *The Basic Fault*—gradually comes to describe a condition prior to Klein's early paranoid-schizoid position, with its projections and splits. In this prior state there is an emptiness that predates envy, the patient being empty of internal objects, whatever their affective colourings. For Enid, "envy seemed only to arise after feelings of being empty of herself had been overcome (that is, after the patient had acquired a feeling of self) and appeared to be connected with a more advanced stage in development" (E. Balint, 1963b, p. 41).

In the clinical description of her patient Sarah, Enid Balint notes that one of the main themes was the difficulty one person must experience in recognising another: "She could never understand how I should know who she was when I went to the waiting room to fetch her for her session" (ibid., p. 42). This is in line with Michael Balint's theory in *The Basic Fault* of two types of regression: the malignant regression aimed at the gratification of instinctual cravings, and the benign regression aimed at recognition (M. Balint, 1968, p. 144). For Enid, who was attempting to flesh out what this meant in terms of interaction with the infant, an essential early experience is the interactive mechanism between mother and baby that she calls an "echo", or "feedback" (E. Balint, 1963a, p. 478). Winnicott is central to her understanding here, and she developed further his ideas of a good enough mother as an unconscious mental state, regarding an ordinary reciprocity to exist when:

> the infant ... gets to know himself, and his mother at the same time, by how she reacts to him. If the mother's reactions do not make sense to the child because, for instance, she is too preoccupied with her own ideas or feelings, then it is not a proper feed-back. On the other hand, good mothering, or proper feed-back, is what makes sense to the child.
>
> (E. Balint, 1993, p. 55)

By reminding us that there is no such thing as a mother without a baby, Enid Balint asserts the other side of Winnicott's postulate that, considered in isolation, there is no such thing as a baby.

Some patients, whilst having been attended to with some appropriateness at a functional level, have never been imaginatively perceived by their mother. This can leave them living a manageable (if quirky) life, but privately they are alone, or even in a solipsistic state. In childhood, such patients often had the capacity for private work, called play. Such creativity develops as part of unconscious phantasy life, yet, when this is shown forth, either in analysis or in artistic creativity, it can produce agonising fear in the patient or artist in case the experience is lost. There is a dilemma whether or not to portray it, in case it is too overwhelming for the analyst, the audience, or the patient's or artist's own compliant self. Either way chaos, madness, or horror may threaten. The greatest fear, though, always seems to be that the experience cannot be repeated and will be lost.

(ibid., p. 101)

Whilst this is happening in the analysis, the task for the analyst is to not intrude, and to just be quietly there. The analysis will need to go through a period in which the analyst cannot—and must not—be perceived by the patient, only to be an unnoticed existence in the room. Usually, such processes occur with an attentive mother. If this maternal presence has not been sufficient, however, or if there is only a surface veneer of care, the infant has recourse to a place with no object. For Enid Balint, this space is not a void, but rather the space that the infant lives in—a space which is alive, rather than the dead space described by André Green (1986). In time, the patient may begin to realise that they are being imaginatively perceived, and can exist in the eye of the other. For Enid, the infant cannot perceive reality unless it is, at the same time, perceived reciprocally by another. Such reciprocality represents the continuation of creative life beyond that of being alone—or, in Winnicott's language, this progression is one of being able, in time, to make use of the object.

In her paper "Creative Life", Enid takes Alice Balint's direction on early object-relating further: "My idea is that the first imaginative perception can only arise out of a state of eager aliveness in two people, the infant with the potential for life and the mother alive inside herself and tuning in to the emerging infant" (E. Balint, 1989, p. 102). She goes on to place the development of a sense of aliveness in imaginative perception:

The danger in analysis is that the patient may try to repeat this passive, accepting "feed" which the analyst offers by his being there as a person, as well as providing couch, chair, an atmosphere of warmth, interpretations, and so on. It may take a long time, perhaps years, before the patient can take the risk of looking away from the mirror and rejecting the person behind the couch and what he stands for. Then a new phase is entered and new work can start.

(ibid., p. 103)

Here she is describing Balint's "Area of the Basic Fault", which, she goes on to write, can only be overcome

> when the patient is no longer regressed to a stage where he has no mutual experience with his analyst but becomes silently hostile, disillusioned, and desperate and eventually appears to give up hope. He sometimes does this without reproaching the analyst, who may wonder what he is doing wrong. He realises, though, that he must not be passively overwhelmed by the patient's projections, which have to be followed even more minutely than usual, and he must also watch his own rigid expectations. This state is overcome only when the patient painfully allows himself to feel alone, in the analyst's presence but with no *person* being there. He may then be able to perceive for himself and to enter the Area of Creativity. The patient is alone with no other person present, but the space is not empty. There is no experience of a void, and the analytic hour is in fact a relief from the previous experience of compliance. Although bringing no apparent satisfaction, it comes to fill the patient's life. To escape from the state of passivity is satisfying in itself. In order, therefore, to get out of the Area of the Basic Fault, my view is that the Area of Creativity has to be entered.

(ibid., pp. 103–104, italics in original)

This is a description of patients who had no early mutual experience that would enable them to feel at home in the world. For Enid Balint, the types of life that can result as a consequence are either passive acceptance, or rebelliousness and rejection. Such children had often been perceived as frightening objects who might easily die, "so they experienced their mothers and the world in which they were living as full of dread and fear" (ibid., p. 108). For Enid, this is an account of patients who are full of something, albeit negative and hostile. She has also reported the opposite situation—those patients who are empty of themselves, who live in a void, because of the absence of reflection of the external world. Hers is a theoretical description and vision that does justice to patients who live in an impasse, a state of being with the other that is malignant regression—but also a description that can suggest an analytic direction towards health. For Enid the point of an analysis is to find a gap and face the awfulness of seeing it. Such a way has nothing to do with words and may have more to do with the patient realising for the first time that he or she is being seen by the analyst and therefore the analyst exists for the patient. Creativity then is a partial solution that can never alter the original gap. However the energy used in not seeing can be directed towards a creative life. The problem with theory is that it can be a convenient cover up of the gap. Her dislike of Kleinian theory was how often she felt it was misused to form a ready made solution rather than the patient discovering their own for themselves.

Analytic training

Semper reformari debet
—reform unremittingly, the motto of the Unitarian Church of Hungary, quoted at the end of Balint's speech at the 1953 IPA Congress in London.

(M. Balint, 1954, p. 285)

Also interested in psychoanalytic training, Balint wrote a pair of papers on the subject that seem, despite their age, to offer trenchant views still alive today. In some respects, he continued to press Ferenczi's original insistence that:

> Above all, we ourselves must have been really well analyzed, right down to "rock bottom". We must have learnt to recognize all our unpleasant external and internal character traits in order that we may be really prepared to face all those forms of hidden hatred and contempt that can be so cunningly disguised in our patient's associations.

(Ferenczi, 1933, p. 158)

Ferenczi was concerned by the possibility that patients may be better analysed than analysts themselves. This observation eventually led to the formal establishment of a required personal analysis as part of the tripartite psychoanalytic training, which was first established in 1925 in the Berlin Society. Training was established soon after in Vienna, then in Budapest. In the same paper, Ferenczi laid stress on the authenticity of the analyst, and notes various forms of potential professional hypocrisy. It is this theme that motivates Balint's desire for the analyst to be unobtrusive in the clinical encounter.

Balint was an advocate of the Hungarian training, in which the third training case is supervised by the candidate's training analyst—in addition to the usual position of both a male and a female training supervisor for the first two cases. The argument prompting this structure is that, often when the supervising training analyst feels that the supervision is touching on a particular piece of the candidate's countertransference, this difficulty can then be taken into the private space of personal analysis for further engagement. Whether something is achieved or not is often unknown, despite the possibility that the difficulty may touch on something important or even essential for the future analyst to grasp about themselves, in relation to their technique with a particular problem in the transference. With their private knowledge of the unconscious character and traumata of the candidate, the training analyst, as third supervisor, can be particularly helpful in such dark areas of unconscious work.

As this supervision occurs towards the latter part of the candidate's personal analysis, it is hoped that, within the setting of the free associations of the analysis, this additional activity will not interfere with the process. On the contrary, it can lead to the uncovering of deeper layers in the mind of the candidate, the elucidation of which can have a profound impact on present and future analytic work. Often this work examines unconscious sibling relationships, as well as parental, with the material from the training case being heard through such private unconscious prisms. If the particular difficulty that the candidate is experiencing with their training case can be analysed, it can shed light both on their own analysis and on their specific problem with the case.

Summary

For all his clinical and theoretical forcefulness, Balint also had a light touch. The opening chapter of his book *Thrills and Regressions* starts with a description of funfairs and excitement: "the essential human needs they satisfy", he writes, "must stem from rather primitive layers of the mind" (M. Balint, 1959, p. 19). He examines human pleasures that revert back to three fundamental factors: "the objective external danger giving rise to fear, the voluntary and intentional exposure of oneself to it, and the confident hope that all will turn out well in the end" (ibid., p. 24). For this, the knowledge that one has, in the past, been safely held—so that this expectation resides in one's unconscious as a given—is profound. Those who felt let down by their environmental provision in early life profoundly fear the thrills and tumbles in the exploration of a funfair experience. Yet, despite harbouring a profound anxiety that they will be dropped yet again, more often there is a very small piece of hope for the future, despite its dangers. We are back in the terrain of early trauma, environmental failure, and the need to handle regression clinically, with concern. The development of this work was the task that he brought with him to London.

When Balint arrived in London as Ferenczi's "main disciple and successor" (Haynal, 1988, p. xvi), he not only brought with him the theories elaborated by the Budapest School, which he aimed to develop, but was also determined to re-establish Ferenczi's rightful place in analytic history—conscious that the latter's significance had considerably waned since his death in 1933. Ferenczi had had his character defamed by Ernest Jones, an analysand, who had written that, towards his death, he had been mad. To this end, and as the literary inheritor of Ferenczi, he brought with him the clinical diary that Ferenczi had kept during the last months of his life, between January and October 1932. It was the diary that furnished "substantial proof, if any were needed, of Ferenczi's sound mental health" (Dupont, 1988, p. xi).

To return to the start of this chapter, the genesis of Ferenczi's final project resides in an essential need to recap and re-evaluate the clinical and theoretical arguments that he had had with Freud, much of which centred on techniques for dealing with regression. Balint realised not only the considerable historical value of this relationship, but that the correspondence also threw light on a plethora of early psychoanalytic ideas, theories-in-the-making, and clinical values. Balint's goal to publish the correspondence, together with the diary, became his passion. For many years he negotiated with Anna Freud, who had retained Ferenczi's side of the correspondence. He also negotiated with Ferenczi's stepdaughter for permission to publish the letters written by Freud, the unconscious significance of intimate family relationships offering profound insights into the layers of meaning in this great correspondence.

Michael Balint died on the last day of 1970, prior to final publication, but the momentum for this great analytic project continued, Enid Balint and Judith Dupont eventually overseeing the publication of the letters between 1992 and 2000, in addition to Ferenczi's *Clinical Diary*, published in French in 1985, with the English edition following three years later. At the end of the *Diary* one can find Balint's draft introduction. Since May 2012, a large Ferenczi archive, including the diary, is housed in the Freud Museum in London. The archive, originally brought to London by Michael Balint, then looked after by Enid, followed by Judith Dupont, was donated on the sole condition it be made accessible to anyone interested in the life and work of Ferenczi, and in contemporary analysis related to the Budapest School. The psychoanalyst Professor André Haynal, in Geneva, had looked after Balint's extensive personal archive since Enid's death. It was fitting that Balint's papers were returned in 2014 to London, in order to be preserved in the archive of the British Psychoanalytical Society. (There is also a further archive donated by Enid of her and Michael's work and correspondence at the Albert Sloman Library at the University of Essex.) Balint's influence as one of the leading exponents of object relation's theory has been considerable. As a major theoretician in the life of the British Society he secured a new beginning for the further exploration of Hungarian psychoanalysis. Back in London, Ferenczi's diary, Balint's papers, and the Hungarian tradition can be well cared for, nurturing the continuance of that essential strand of independent psychoanalysis. It keeps alive that dialogue and understanding of depth analysis, especially that essential component of countertransference, which not only enriches psychoanalytic understandings of unconscious life but, with Balint's significant contribution to many related fields, also furthers knowledge in psychosomatics, regression, general medicine, and teaching.

CHAPTER TWO

Training and supervision: between learning technique and developing authenticity

Maybe the moment hasn't arrived yet.
Let's not be too hasty: haste is a dangerous thing.
Untimely measures bring repentance.
Certainly, and unhappily, many things in the Colony are
absurd.
But is there anything human without some fault?
And after all, you see, we do move forward.

—C. P. Cavafy, *"In a Large Greek Colony, 200 BC"* (1928)

Perhaps then one reason why we have no great poet, novelist or critic
writing to-day is that we refuse words their liberty. We pin them down to
one meaning, their useful meaning, the meaning which makes us catch the
train, the meaning which makes us pass the examination.

—Virginia Woolf, *"Craftsmanship"* (1937)

In modern times I will argue that there are both external and internal ways that psychoanalytic training can be impeded, and also that this is perhaps inevitable. We will examine the early formations of analytical training and how external rules on how best to practise and evaluate the profession displaced the analyst's own internalised authority. And we will explore the form of the analytic setting in relation to the specific analytic psychic dimension of the analyst and analysand being in the consulting room together—currently being threatened by the new mode of video call and phone analysis. More generally, we will consider the importance of fostering an elasticity of technique both in analysis and in its training.

An external agency can attempt to control training from outside of the profession, such as a determination to introduce stringent rules of governance—aimed more perhaps at controlling a system than arising from a concern for efficacy, ethics, or the understanding of unconscious processes. An example in the UK would be the NHS: how it attempts to offer therapy for the masses via brief cognitive therapy, or just six sessions of psychotherapy, and how it expects the same models for developing professionalism and skills in such settings to be acceptable for examining the complexities of psychoanalysis. Such matters are less about the good training of therapists than settling on a cheap model with the short-term goal of quick, cost-effective treatments. Unfortunately, many patients revert swiftly back to their ill states of mind. Most patients referred to me for a consultation have already had their six sessions or so of treatment, which have proved ineffectual in treating their complex material.

Psychoanalytic societies also develop systems of regulation, with educational committees developing rules and procedures in an attempt to organise measuring tools and enhance the quality of training. These matters have a history that goes as far back as the beginning of formal analytic training, to the establishment of the original Berlin training in 1920 by Max Eitingon, Karl Abraham, and Ernst Simmel, and the progressive formalisation of their regulations. Prior to that there were no particular formalities or theories about supervision and training. Beginning in 1902, Freud held weekly evening meetings in his apartment in which theory and clinical work would be presented and discussed with colleagues and friends. In 1908, when the Vienna Psychoanalytic Society was formed, this loose circle became a functional meeting of the new Society. From 1910, *"everyone who attended the meetings was required to participate in the discussions"* (H. Nunberg, 1959, italics in original). Later, in both his seminars and Balint groups, Balint was also famous for inviting everyone in the circle, at a certain point, to give an opinion on a case, perhaps basing this on Freud's demand. It is worth quoting

Herman Nunberg on the sort of interests of those early meetings at Freud's apartment: "Papers were read, books and magazine articles were reviewed ... biology, animal psychology, psychiatry, sociology, mythology, religion, art and literature, education and criminology" (ibid., p. xxii). It is useful to remember, in relation to today's debates about the necessary contents of analytic training, that the beginnings of group consideration of psychoanalysis focused on ideas from such wide-ranging fields. At that time there was no formal requirement to have an analysis as part of training. This only became established following insistent pressure from Ferenczi, who confronted the analytic community with the conundrum that a problematic split would develop in which analysands would become better analysed than the cadre of analysts. This realisation would lead to the establishment of analytic training in Berlin, and to making training analysis the bedrock in the formation of the analytic candidate.

The first training guidelines were issued from Berlin in 1924 (M. Balint, 1947, p. 257). The analysis of the student analyst was considered essential, initially lasting at least six months. Trainees had to complete two years of supervised clinical treatment in Berlin. Two years later, the Vienna Society issued its own training rules, doubling the training requirements set out in Berlin, and requiring two supervisors and four cases for those training in Vienna. The analyst of the trainee did not function at the same time as the supervisor to their training analysand, the two parts of the training being kept separate in order to maintain the privacy and boundary of the analysis. By contrast, in the third centre in Budapest, it was encouraged that trainees were supervised on their third case by their own analyst, acting in a double role. The rationale behind this was that the supervisor-analyst would be in a unique position to recognise and speak to that part of the trainee-patient that was struggling with their countertransference to their own patient. Otherwise, when the candidate was in clinical difficulty due to their own conflicts and defences, all the supervisor could do in the other models was to suggest that the candidate presented the issue in their separate, private analysis. Such suggestion could be either taken up or ignored—in the privacy of the candidate's own desires for their analysis.

The point of these descriptions of the early training methods is twofold. Within a couple of years of the first establishment of formal training, different national schemes began increasing the training requirements.

This can be seen as a development of the process of regulation, but it can also be viewed as the beginning of a competition to be regarded as more competent and more rigorous. In addition, significant differences began to emerge surrounding the complexity of analysis and its impact on training. After a few years there were several forms of analytic training, each of which stood on its own empirical platform, as well as being embedded in a particular local culture. Already, this first divergence of trainings is a leap from Freud's thought that the analyst "can [not 'ought to', or even 'should'] get supervision and guidance from recognized psycho-analysts" (Freud, 1919j, p. 171). The debate had already shifted from the need for training centred on the candidate to a discussion more concerned with particular conventions—and even doctrines—in the training committee.

By the mid-1930s, more intensive discussion about the rationale of such practices had begun, and it has long continued. For many years the European Psychoanalytic Federation (EPF) has held an annual Forum on Education, where an established group of experienced colleagues present to each other on their supervision of analytic candidates—within the boundaries of confidentiality. The complexity of the multi-layered encounters which are examined ranges from between the trainee analyst and their patient, onto the supervisor–supervisee complex, and then along the supervisor–institution axis. Everyone participating in the conference comes from their own analytic tradition, which may be similar or radically different from other European colleagues. Teaching psychoanalysis has become more complex but perhaps also narrower and less direct than Freud's approach in Vienna—a narrowing resulting from a conflict between the candidate's preoccupation with both requirements and evaluations and the maintenance of a free-floating atmosphere in which they can learn about unconscious process. Having a training system also invites some analysts to evaluate how the training functions too frequently, constantly pursuing a goal of discerning the best methods—a Sisyphean task similar to evaluating a "best" unconscious.

* * *

To understand more of what is at stake here, we need go beyond the 1930s and Balint's papers of the 1940s, onto the 1950s. In 1952, Siegfried Bernfeld gave a paper named "On Psychoanalytic Training" to the San Francisco Society—although this was not published until 1962. Bernfeld trained in analysis with Freud in Vienna from around 1919 through the early 1920s. In 1937 he immigrated to the US, settling in San Francisco. His paper explored the sense of freedom of his early analytic training prior to the establishment of psychoanalytic training institutes, along with his concern about models of teaching and authority in the institute. As time passes, this paper shows little sign of dating, and can still be read as an invitation to reconsider the interesting problems always bedevilling analytic training and its institutionalisation. Bernfeld is decidedly on the side of the process of analytic education rather than its organisation, early in the paper postulating the idea of "free institutions" in order to counteract what he perceives as the dangers of institutionalisation. In the introduction to the published paper we are told that some colleagues thought his convictions on training stemmed from his feelings that discussions with his local education committee had been fruitless, leading him to resign from it. He was not preoccupied by being piqued by colleagues, however; he was concerned for the future development of psychoanalysis. His paper, far from being restricted in scope to his observations of that one American analytic society, applies to all analytic training. As Rudolf Ekstein describes in an introduction to the paper, Bernfeld is interested in what he called student-centred (rather than teacher-centred) learning, and, in particular, with the spirit of psychoanalysis, rather than "administrative considerations, struggles about minimum requirements, admissions policies, etc." (Bernfeld, 1962, p. 455).

We can make a link here to a book in which the EPF Working Party on Comparative Clinical Methods proposed a new framework specifically to look at certain supervision questions (Tuckett, 2008). As Arne Jemstedt writes in his chapter on their research, "The aim was to minimize the risk of a situation where discussion in the group would be obscured by difficulties or impasses in the work being explored" (Jemstedt, 2008, p. 78). Meanwhile, David Tuckett argues that: "'Free discussion' had significant drawbacks. We have subsequently learnt that a degree of structure can be useful whenever psychoanalysts discuss clinical material" (Tuckett, 2008, p. 134). This is an interesting experiment, but its formality at once pitches itself away from a core Freudian position of unconscious communication that knows no rules and does not recognise such structure. Similarly, in an analytic session, if one is looking out for a specific thing, then one is far from the mindset of being available as a free listener. The same is true of supervisory material. When articulating his concern for analytic process over structure, Bernfeld pointed out a pattern that continues to inevitably emerge as a more conscious attempt to frame and perhaps tame the difficulties or impasses in the work. Writing from a similar perspective, in a discussion in *The Freudian Moment* of the high value that Freud placed on free association, Christopher Bollas argues, "Look not for what you think is the most exalted, but examine the apparently trivial or the irrelevant" (Bollas, 2007, p. 12). This is a valuing of the individual idiom of each analyst, and works in tune with Freud's concept of the analyst as a particular receiver for the patient's unconscious material. The greater the attempts to categorise speech or topics in particular analytic encounters, the remoter the possibility of ambling along without interference to see where the next moment takes us. The skein of free associations can quickly disappear, allowing us to forget that, for anyone engaged in trying to reach the unconscious, free association really matters.

This is not to ignore how hard it is to teach the ideal analytic procedure that Freud describes, in his "Two Encyclopaedia Articles", as a form of "surrender":

> Experience soon showed that the attitude which the analytic physician could most advantageously adopt was to surrender himself to his own unconscious mental activity, in a state of *evenly suspended attention*, to avoid so far as possible reflection and the construction of conscious expectations, not to try to fix anything that he heard particularly in his memory, and by these means to catch the drift of the patient's unconscious with his own unconscious.

> (Freud, 1923a, p. 239, italics in original)

And if such an attitude cannot be taught, then it is vital in supervision that, at the very least, an atmosphere centred on this unusual approach can be allowed to subsist as something of analytic value. When attempting to evaluate the analytic functioning of a candidate or colleague, we have the problem of what to understand by the "acts of speech" in which the analytical experience is described. When presented, descriptions of past sessions require an ability to communicate atmosphere and experience, and so if language is not up to the task of describing the, at times, enduring internal horror (as it often is not), then how is one to do this without words? I use such a strong word because the reader will have come across descriptions of horror that occur regularly in clinical analytic life, and which even in reading can elicit strong feelings of revulsion. Unconscious communication between the analyst and analysand can utilise silent affect. As words find their way to the surface an eruption of involuntary memory may occur (in a Proustian sense) which cuts through the other sentences and allows the emergence of the unthought known. The supervisor needs to proceed with care to enable this found object to live, as it can be as quick to burst as the disappearance of the dream on the sudden awakening of the dreamer.

Bernfeld's position on the periphery of the institution, as a lecturer and analyser of candidates, bears analogy to collegiate meetings of European psychoanalysts, where representatives from many psychoanalytic societies—with both similar and quite different trainings—meet independently of their institutions. Such conference work is outside of the superstructures of each society and their particular educational policies. From such an outside position, investigations on training can be pursued with a degree of freedom precisely because one is invited to be and to think from an unusual position, outside of one's own society. Informality and a relative absence of institutional transferences can open up unconscious space for thinking. This is one of the abiding aspects of the usefulness of the EPF, the accent falling away from the specific dogma and culture of the individual society. Sometimes one needs to move away for a while in order to see more clearly that which is under our nose every day. More analytic societies are developing, especially in the east of the European region, with all their mixtures of the cultural and traumatic histories of the twentieth century. Instead of being pulled towards propounding a particular type of theory (a way of avoiding the complex milieu of analytic theories), an immersion in a European analytic culture and structure that values difference, and enables discussion around difficult edges, can make a huge difference to how an individual analyst thinks in the wider field. Bernfeld argued that:

> The training that is conducted in our professional schools distorts some of the most valuable features of psychoanalysis and hinders its development as a science and as a tool by means of which to change behavior ... My statements that the institutes carry out their training obligations but, on the other hand, that they are detrimental to psychoanalysis may seem contradictory; yet the paradox simply

expresses one of the most important insights of the psychoanalytic theory of education.

(Bernfeld, 1962, pp. 458–459)

We do need a structure to administer the complexities of training. But we must be careful. For instance, Laplanche and Pontalis (1967, p. 89) describe the candidate's analysis, instituted in 1920, as "control analysis". The word "control" has a negative connotation in the English language, in conflict with the need for candidates to have the freedom of mind necessary for understanding their own unconscious process. Nowadays such a term is rarely used, yet it still exists, more under the surface and unconsciously available for candidate, analyst, and training committee. To know, befriend, and ultimately, through insight, to have some sway over one's passions is perhaps a better description than the ambiguity of the term "control". Of course, the candidate needs to control their passions, and this can be one of the difficulties of maintaining an analytic attitude at the same time as the idiomatic character, as Bollas would say, of the individual analyst themselves.

Using an argument about school education, Bernfeld suggests that many forms of education lead to learning, but not all subsequently ensure growth and development following the end of the training period. The more authoritarian the training, the less love of analytic learning later. One can certainly see such potential dynamics in many analytic societies. Some societies add more tasks "for the good of the training" that, viewed from the candidate's side, become additional burdens to overcome before reaching the finishing line. It is hard not to notice the conflict between the training managers that want finer and better learning modules (as they see it) and the candidates' feelings that these strictures curtail the freedom of an ideal training—one with an atmosphere of openness, and a pleasure taken in the work and its developments.

* * *

Today we are confronted with the same issues in a new form when, for example, we face pressure to ensure that the standards of analytic training are available for external scrutiny as well as evaluation. Government-appointed committees or insurance companies who have little knowledge of, and even less use for unconscious process have become interested in our trainings. Much of this is in relation to burgeoning non-analytical psychotherapy models. Government, whilst speaking about protecting the general public from untrained or rogue therapists, has another agenda of producing structures to contain the development of brief treatment models that cost less, on the surface, than psychoanalysis or analytic psychotherapy. It also wishes to evaluate the psychoanalytic model through the same prism, requiring a manualised account of treatment and asking for patient feedback in the same way as asking if a hospital was clean and friendly. Asking for patient feedback from an analysand in treatment is an interference in the daily work and may well alter depending on whether the question is asked on a Monday or a Friday. The daily residue is no respecter of questionnaires.

Many new procedures are being introduced into the psychological professions. These new standards and requirements often soon reveal themselves to be ways of controlling professional life. For some, the quest for a manual of analytic practice promises the simplification of the training task, allowing the simplicity of ticking the analyst's utterances as either correct or incorrect, as a way of "really knowing" their work. In a similar fashion, some candidates might prefer the simplicity of a how-to manual, including the sort of interpretation that may be made when the patient says particular things. I would argue that this more reflects a wish to stay on the surface of clinical material, and can indicate a profound anxiety—on the part of the patient, but sometimes more so in the candidate—about the unconscious beneath.

A new form of social control over psychotherapy is being developed in the UK by the Department of Health, using what it calls "key performance indicators" in describing therapy. The targets are more concerned with numbers than with people. Unsurprisingly, one of the measurements of such a programme's success is the number of people that can be removed from financial benefits. At each and every session, clients are asked a series of standard questions by the therapist in order to generate figures that are taken to represent a level of anxiety or depression. Such numbers go into a database, along with details of any employment or benefit status. Gathering positive scores, or at least appearing to get better, may mean keeping one's job. Anyone with a modicum of knowledge, however, knows that anxious or depressed people sometimes do not accurately report their own experience. So here we have a government department examining data with a vested interest to control the therapeutic field in very specific ways. If this means generating false data, such as asking the patient to rate each session (as an exercise apparently separate from the clinical work done only a few moments earlier), then its clinical implications, not least in the transference and the fact that this effectively means setting up a control system inside the therapy, are presumably supposed to be ignored.

As Darian Leader argues in "Some Thoughts on Supervision":

> Now that the government has recognized the value of talking therapies and set itself the task of guaranteed service provision within a set time period for those judged to be in need, the only mechanism which would make this goal possible is a deskilling of the workforce. As psychology graduates and even students are brought in to offer rudimentary "therapy", so the role of the more fully trained—and much more expensive—therapists becomes subtly pushed towards group supervision rather than direct practice. This is arguably one aspect of the future for therapists working in many NHS trusts.
>
> (Leader, 2010, p. 229)

Continuing his argument, Leader shows how destructive such external control will be in our professional life:

> It also implies that therapists will spend more and more time supervising trainee clinicians who have had no analysis or therapy themselves, a problem that is currently being widely debated. This is crucial to the question of supervision since, once we assume that the supervisee has not embarked on the self-exploratory journey of a talking therapy him- or herself, supervision starts to swing in precisely the direction that the regulatory literature has taken. Once unconscious dynamics are deemed peripheral, all that is left is the knowledge and skills model of supervision in which the supervisor becomes almost responsible for the trainee's clinical work. This suggests that any critique of this model of supervision must also insist on the centrality of the experience of personal analysis or therapy for the trainee. And isn't this, after all, exactly what defines our field of the talking therapies?
>
> (ibid., p. 229)

Leader is describing the marginalisation of the psychoanalytic experience by national regulation. However, psychoanalysis as both treatment and training, and in its embrace by academia, remains a central component of human knowledge. In the UK, as well as throughout both Europe and the US, psychiatry, regarding itself as scientific, has distanced itself from psychoanalysis, having a psychoanalytic training often being seen as a disadvantage to becoming a consultant in the NHS. However, this has left analysis free to grow separately over the many years, and without political distractions. Psychiatry in the new century, realising the benefit of enlarging the reach of counselling services, now desires a sort of "psychoanalysis-lite" as part of its domain. By accepting such a development, the analytic profession will be required to be more externally controlled. But the essence of unconscious processes and free association is intrinsically incompatible with any such frame.

British psychoanalysis, never at the centre of psychiatry (unlike in the US for many decades up until the 1970s), now finds itself being pushed even further outside of recognised orthodoxy. Whilst some may despair at such a rejection of the standards specific to psychoanalytic practice, there is another way of looking at these developments. Unconscious processes in analytic treatment, necessarily under the surface, might now need to include an acceptance that to be at the centre of a healthcare plan or insurance scheme requires admitting a third party to the privacy of the analytic couple. Many insurance schemes, in particular the German and Dutch state systems, allow each citizen a certain number of sessions of analysis per year of free treatment. These sessions have been paid for by the state. Yet regular and full reports are expected, a light description that "analytic work was done" not deemed sufficient. Confidentiality as a value therefore disappears. Superficially, this may seem to suggest that the analyst is being given wider social recognition, but this is at a price. Confidential material has to be regularly shared with the insurance company or the state, making a mockery of the idea of privacy. In the unconscious, the knowledge of the fact that the third party knows and receives regular accounts of something or other of the intimate work has its own effect. As the years pass, new candidates develop their practice completely inside of such a welfare system, knowing only by distant hearsay how confidentiality in analysis used to be sacred. The implication in the present analytic unconscious today is that leakage is to be expected. Regular reports on treatments are given and cannot be evaded. If we are not careful, after many years they might come to be regarded as the norm. And so perhaps being outside such governmental nets—whilst seeming to give psychoanalysis a lower societal status, and even lower fees—can provide a safer place for the pursuit of the privacy of the analytic dyad. Even a government agency knowing the name or social security number of our patients is interference. Some might respond by asking what should happen when an analysand wants to claim costs from their private insurance. Here my response would be that it would be their own decision, but also that, if they choose such a path of financial support, then it would be odd if their treatment had to be curtailed by a junior clerk, with no clinical experience, imposing budget-imposed limits. Such an external rupture is completely at odds with the analysand's need to be the one who authorises their own treatment.

* * *

These are some of the minefields that await our profession if we put ourselves in the hands of external regulators. Yet the problem also exists inside the institutes of psychoanalysis. For Bernfeld, some of our own analytic educational structures can function in similar ways—existing to reify a particular theoretical model, for example, or becoming part of an underlying political situation within a society. Bernfeld trenchantly notes in his paper that those of us with particular views—"partisans", as he calls us—cannot be easily argued with. We need to be alert to the unconscious determinants of institutional processes. In relation to this, he considers the 1922 diagnosis of Freud's cancer to have been crucial to the body of psychoanalysts:

> I need not explain in detail what Freud's "death and resurrection" within this one year meant to the older psychoanalysts in Vienna and Berlin ... [Some] grew intensely anxious because of the threatened loss, and became very eager to establish a solid dam against heterodoxy, as they now felt themselves responsible for the future of psychoanalysis. They determined to limit by rigid selection among the newcomers, and by the institution of a coercive, long drawn-out trial period of authoritarian training, any final admission to their societies. In fact, they punished their students for their own ambivalence. At the same time, they consolidated the one trend that Freud always had wanted to avoid: the shrinkage of psychoanalysis into an annex of psychiatry.
>
> (Bernfeld, 1962, p. 467)

Such profound unconscious resonances are not of course only specific to Freud and his immediate successors. German candidates today also have to notice how their societies handle psychoanalysis, the Holocaust, and the past authority of the Nazis. In an Anglo-German colloquium, some years ago German analysts spoke with much dismay about their often having great difficulty to speak up with an "analytic authority" as they felt disqualified by the burden of their history. Other societies have their own painful history and historical context that constitute part of an unconscious culture. This may be due to war, the ending of communist hegemony, or splits due to personal animosities. Such matters can stay submerged for many long years within the culture of an analytic society, yet be tripped over by candidates.

Such anxieties can be seen at work in the question of who should be an analyst. In 1927 at the International Psycho-analytical Association (IPA) Innsbruck Congress, a decision was made to disallow lay candidates of the North American Region from the training and practice of analysis. The year before, Freud had published "A Question of Lay Analysis" (1926e), a passionate and well-argued defence against such obstacles to training. Despite Freud's intervention, the rule allowing only medically trained analysts in the US was only rescinded in 1988. As early as 1920, Freud had written to Abraham: "I am tremendously pleased that things are so active in Berlin, and that you too are now beginning to be convinced of the impossibility of restricting psychoanalysis to the doctors" (21 June 1920; Freud, 1965a, p. 312).

The atmosphere engendered by the premonition of Freud's death, followed by his resurrection, may still be unconsciously available to societies today. After all, we all have our icons. For London they are Sigmund Freud, Anna Freud, Klein, Balint, Winnicott, and Bion. Such treasures are still fought over. In London, in May 2005, following a vote at the British Society, administrative regulation via the three theoretical groups ceased, bringing an end to the so called Gentlemen's Agreement that had kept the Society together following the Controversial Discussions of the 1940s. In 1946, the Freudian, Kleinian, and independent analysts had agreed to an unwritten rule that there would be representatives of all three "groups" on the main committees of the society—that is, the council, the training committee, and other policymaking bodies. No group would be able to be eliminated by another group, and unity was maintained despite diversity (King & Steiner, 1991, p. 907). Over many years, one of the groups (the Contemporary Freudians, as the Anna Freud group had become known) became very small, whilst another expanded its percentage of training analysts (the Kleinian group). Arguably, this made it difficult for the tripartite representation to continue being maintained on the important education committees. With one group being much larger in number, a formal vote to disband the unwritten constitution was easily won. Although nobody prevented colleagues from meeting privately in groups, the slogan became "Groups have now ceased". A monitoring system was set up to ensure a balanced training across the three different theoretical modes—politics and power, however, can dominate behind such surface appearances. Like the tension between manifest and latent, a double rhetoric developed, consciously paying attention to divergences in the group, but unconsciously discouraging difference. Ten years on there was no monitoring. Any potential training applicant, not knowing about recent political schisms, may not understand that their desire to be in treatment with a particular analysis, or their wish to train predominantly in one of the theoretical groups, may be thwarted by the surface mantra that "all training analysts are now members of the British Society", which has magically eradicated the differences from the three groups. Groups are abolished, yet they continue (another death and resurrection). Such matters can pose ethical problems around what a candidate knows, what they ought to know, and what they should be informed about at the start of an analysis. The analyst from a now apparently deceased group cannot suddenly reframe themselves away from their theoretical internal objects to become group-free. Such new political structures can stand in the way of a discovery of self that is free from such contamination. Profound disagreement in theory, instead of being debated, is now often regarded as having been resolved by the new joined-up society. Diffidence towards the other's theoretical and clinical practices can trickle down from on high to be reflected in some candidates' naïve and irrational disdain for analytical views other to those of their analyst. These occurrences in analytic societies expose the passivity of intellectual rigour and the paucity of debate. None of this is news. The IPA is full of societies that have had to split because of intangible as well as obvious disagreements. Often it comes down to the use or perceived use of power, or to differences between strong characters. Somehow candidates have to navigate such difficult terrain, beneath the surface of the training.

Once the hurdle of training has been overcome the next obstacle then presents itself, with new and more specific rules and regulations about becoming a senior member or fellow. It is easily argued that it is for the good of analytic competency or, as perceived by recently qualified associates, that more and more training demands are needed—the old issue of the primal horde. The problem is not so much in the details of such postgraduate programmes but in the experience of young colleagues within their system. For many, continuing training after qualification is not worth bothering with. Bernfeld signalled this when describing how authoritarian learning leads to the pupil not enjoying further learning when an adult, as noted earlier. Perhaps to progress professionally in analytic societies requires a particular form of not knowing about the negative aspects of collegiate life. How can training institutes renew themselves from their often very weighty baggage, then? One answer would be that by temporarily leaving our home to meet colleagues with perhaps different views on analysis, training, and authority, we can realise again that our own institutional way is not perhaps the way of the true cross. From a deep knowledge of our personal history and our historical culture, the analyst can, in time, form their own authority and authenticity towards the analytic function.

As an example of an area in which it has been necessary to challenge an institutional line or development, let us examine an issue at the heart of analytic training. I will quote a letter sent to all European society presidents by Laurence Kahn and Patrick Miller:

> We would like to express our deep concern about an IPA policy on "remote analysis" approved by the (IPA) board in July 2009. Conversations between an analyst and a patient on the phone or using Skype, however useful they may be in certain circumstances, should not be called "analysis" when, in the same paragraph, the IPA reassesses that a pre-condition for the analytic method is that "analyst and patient be present in the same room". If this policy were to be included in the Procedural Code we fear that it would have a disastrous effect on training and hence on the future of analysis. It is the IPA's role to defend the specificity of the analytic method and to protect it from degradation for opportunistic reasons.
>
> (personal communication, July 2009)

Here, the political desire to expand the field of analysis across the map of the world, like some latter-day Cortés, is seen to have a significant cost for an authentic in-the-consulting-room engagement of unconscious process. To take one detail, the significance of silence in an analysis is profound for all that is not said but felt, in that state of shared quietness. Telephony does not necessarily transmit bundles of silence, as transportation of sound is an expensive commodity. Silence does not travel down the line and instead a signal is sent that is reconstituted at the receiving end as an electronic "silence", one devoid of the humanness that began it. And so, listening to silence on the phone may well interfere with the receiver's unconscious reception. There is no need to make an even more obvious argument against so-called analysis by email. Such apparently progressive developments can lead away from the unconscious commitment to analysis, and are far removed from the following formula of Freud's:

> [The analyst] must turn his own unconscious like a receptive organ towards the transmitting unconscious of the patient. He must adjust himself to the patient as a telephone receiver is adjusted to the transmitting microphone. Just as the receiver converts back into sound waves the electric oscillations in the telephone line which were set up by sound waves, so the doctor's unconscious is able, from the derivatives of the unconscious which are communicated to him, to reconstruct that unconscious, which has determined the patient's free association.
>
> (Freud, 1912e, pp. 115–116)

Freud is talking about vibrating sounds, miniscule registers of affect, the most intangible yet physical resonances that pass in the consulting room from analyst to analysand, and vice versa. The analytic couple being in the same room together is the optimum condition for our work. In addition, learning psychoanalysis is considerably harder when an essential authentic listening component is absent, unable to contribute to the reverie of unconscious communication. One can also speculate on whether the absence of meaningful silence, unless found in some other place, leads to a diminution of unconscious listening after the completion of such a training. I take issue with telephony in relation to psychoanalytic training as it can alter transference and countertransference experience, and the development of the listening ear of the candidate. When it comes to treatment I am aware that many patients lead peripatetic lives, and that if there is no possibility of regularly and frequently being in the consulting room then they would be deprived of a valuable treatment.

I am thinking of businessmen who travel for their work, pilots, and foreign correspondents (there are many other categories). I think it is essential that as much as possible of the clinical work takes place in the consulting room, particularly at the beginning of treatment—thereafter, flexibility in the use of phone analysis can be examined and applied, towards the form of holding, as there is a profound difference between using the couch and having less intimate phone sessions. I am remembering the treatment of a journalist who had to be stationed for several weeks at a time in Baghdad during the Iraq War. His vivid telling over the phone of the intense fear for his life and of the atmosphere of terror probably helped ward off a breakdown when he returned to the UK, where he could benefit from the more usual holding of the consulting room. Yet that piece of near-emergency work had in the background the memory of the intimacy and holding capacity of the couch and consulting room, activated over the line from the violence and fear in Baghdad. In general, the issue of phone or email analysis presents a clear example of the crucial necessity of being able to take a critical stance towards the institutions that regulate our work.

It is all too easy to characterise analysts trying to hold on to the Freudian model, with its emphasis on unconscious process, as unchanging luddites. Of course, theory needs to move away from static knowledge, but this does not mean that the next theoretical move is always valuable or persuasive—as if all radical shifts in psychoanalytic thinking must be a good thing, when they may in fact just reflect an already existing distribution of power and authority inside the institution. Part of the problem is that many candidates ingratiate themselves with a present institutional authority. This may have something to do with the candidate's character, with the analytic power of particular groups, or with the high profile of some training analysts. Despite their own analysis, some analysts may not really want to think too much for themselves, preferring to align themselves with a strong group as an easier option. We all know that free thinking is hard.

Bernfeld is acerbic when he states that "in psychoanalysis, as elsewhere, institutionalization does not encourage thinking" (Bernfeld, 1962, p. 468). Ideally, supervision is an intermediate space between the analysis and the seminar. It is a place where technique—and different types of technique—can be described, discussed, and left open for the candidate to make use of. This is different from a didactic and controlling supervisory experience where one goes to be told how to do analysis technically. There is a great psychological difference between being told how to do something and finding it out for oneself in the presence of the other. The implications of this for the candidate's later work connects with Bernfeld's ideas surrounding the type of teacher and the aftermath of the educational process (that an authoritarian teaching style discourages later learning). That is, if, re-enacting a didactic teaching method, we are convinced we know the right way to do something, then we do not tolerate uncertainty. This is profoundly different to rediscovering in the moment. If one starts from the premise of not knowing, however, then the analyst, throughout their career in the consulting room, always needs to find new ways of learning in order to follow the patient.

Supervision is not analysis, yet the supervisor notices or is invited to see beyond the clinical encounter something about the privateness of the candidate—or how the candidate is or is not accessible and available for the patient to make use of. We are all aware of such complexities, and the candidate is often looking for authority in the training—the correct way—indicating a desire to "join the club". In supervision, the thoughtful supervisor can understand different ways of listening. One can, of course, argue the opposite: that the candidate is attending in order to learn the supervisor's particular model. The supervisory encounter develops the atmosphere of how the supervisor works, with their own openness or rigidities. At the first supervision, Winnicott would take the candidate into the kitchen and make them a cup of tea or coffee, and would say that the next time they might make their own—a light and evocative version of his idea of the use of an object. If the supervisor has a humility about their practice, and a realisation that analysis, complex as it is, has a variety of ways of moving on from any one point in the particular session's material, then this allows a similar mobility in the candidate, who can then find their own love of doing this work with the other, embracing the psychic pain and difficulties of uncertainty, rather than trying to control them.

In her introductory address, "Candidates: Obstacles in the Process of Supervision", at the 2006 EPF Forum on Education in Budapest, Marie-France Dispaux pointed out a current direction of the state of the training itself. Not only does training bring out the oedipal and narcissistic problems of trainees, but also:

> The other challenge encountered by the Supervisor is his function
> as evaluator and this is the role of supervision in the institutional

setting. The institution can be a good third party, a guarantee for both parties, preventing too much idealisation and providing other models of how to go about things ... But the institutional body can also present a burden as much for the supervisor as for the trainee, in inhibiting creativity and originality of thought. Nevertheless, neither one, nor the other—supervisor or trainee—escapes the necessity of evaluation.

(Dispaux, 2006)

How the institution is functioning at the given period in which a person is training undoubtedly colours that training, and even its supervisory material. The candidate may have to ascertain if their supervision is on this or that side of a political divide or a given theoretical set of views. It is quite often variable who has chosen the supervisor: the candidate, the analyst, or the progress advisor. This will have its own place in the unconscious of the candidate.

Supervision can contain acts that go some way to undoing a candidate's repression in relation to their clinical work. This may expose a lacuna in the candidate's own private analysis as something as yet unanalysed, or a piece of resistance in the candidate. This is a very delicate area that cannot be contained by sets of rules, and it requires respect for an evaluation of the process in the candidate's work. If this is undertaken in as open and mutual a way as possible, then even the evaluation will be an activity of tact—an aspect of that being with the other that the clinical work demands. Here the concept of "tact" is taken from Ferenczi's original idea in his 1928 paper "The Elasticity of Psychoanalytic Technique": "The analyst, like an elastic band, must yield to the patient's pull, but without ceasing to pull in his own direction, so long as one position or the other has not been conclusively demonstrated to be untenable" (Ferenczi, 1928, p. 95). A colleague to whom Ferenczi showed the paper for criticism wrote, "The title ['Elasticity'] is excellent ... and should be applied more widely, for Freud's technical recommendations were essentially negative" (ibid., p. 99). This interlocutor was none other than Freud himself, who continued: "Rules for making these measurements can naturally not be made; the analyst's experience and normality will have to be the decisive factors. But one should thus divest 'tact' of its mystical character" (4 January 1928; Freud, 2000, p. 332). The warning to beware rules in relation to clinical work is clear, even if it means that the evaluation tasks of the educational committee are based more on impressionistic than scientific knowledge.

* * *

As an analogy for what I have been describing here, let me quote the English artist Leon Kossoff describing his early supervision in painting classes: "Coming to Bomberg's class was like coming home" (Moorhouse, 1996, p. 12). In David Bomberg he found a liberating presence that confirmed rather than directed the future development of his art. As he recalled: "The life room at St. Martin's at that time was very rigid and inhibiting and I remember a feeling of relief and excitement when I first entered Bomberg's class. People were working in a way I'd only previously dared to work on my own" (ibid.). Despite the force of Bomberg's convictions and personality his classes remained open and free, indeed one of his strengths as a teacher being his sensitivity to the individual needs of different students: "What David did for me which was more important than any technique he could have taught me, was he made me feel I could do it. I came to him with no belief in myself whatsoever and he treated my work with respect" (ibid.). Although this is a description of a different type of supervision, the atmosphere in which the supervisor treats the supervisee is striking. It is important not to romanticise such a position, but for both to be able to respect each other, as well as the working couple. Supervision itself can be a new experience of relating, differing from the early experiences of one's own history. The asymmetry of knowledge and the differing positions between supervisor and supervised require respect from both sides, and the use of tact. Otherwise, one is back in the realms of the problem of power between a junior and a senior colleague. The supervisory experience makes use of a potential space in the mind of the supervisor. At some point, the candidate will find ways of working with the paradox of seeing the supervisor as the keeper of functional knowledge while realising that the validity of that knowledge is less about the particular directions discussed than the realisation of a freedom of thought—of the great possibilities inherent in the ability to pursue many different directions with the patient, as well as with themselves.

It seems obvious to the training organisation that all the rules and procedures have one purpose: to regulate the qualification of analyst. In this position, everything stems from the fact that the authority is vested in the organisation and then bestowed onto the candidate. Whilst that invokes pleasure and relief, the new analyst is often left with intense dilemmas: although they are now an analyst, they are still aware that unconscious process may not be sufficiently available to their own pre-conscious, other than having an external paper certificate that describes them as now being an analyst. In time, the analyst needs to take their own authority that they are an analyst for and as themselves, a process that concerns the internal state of mind of the analyst, alone with them-selves, and free from their own analyst, supervisors, and institution, within the freedom of their own unconscious. The topics discussed here concern both the external regulation of psychoanalysis as well as the history of its internal regulation. The avoidance of both over-regulation and institutionalisation is a profound task that analysts, as members of psychoanalytic institutes, need to maintain vigilance over, in order to maintain freedom and the capacity for free association in both analy-sis and training. There will always be the inevitable presence of poli-tics and power dynamics in both analytic societies and the supervisory experience, and these will always have their impact on candidates and their training. Being aware of such matters decreases the likelihood that the worst is unconsciously enacted—that training analysis relies on mimesis and on emulating the training analyst. It is the first step to ensuring a culture that allows the analyst to find their own authority, in a consulting room of their own.

PART II

BALINT GROUPS

CHAPTER THREE

Balint groups: a history

Landscapes can be deceptive. Sometimes a landscape seems to be less a setting for the life of its inhabitants than a curtain behind which their struggles, achievements and accidents take place. For those who, with the inhabitants, are behind the curtain, landmarks are no longer only geographic but also biographical and personal.

—John Berger, *A Fortunate Man: The Story of a Country Doctor*
(1967, p. 19)

Introduction

Balint groups are a way of extending the understanding of unconscious states of mind into the atmosphere of ordinary medical practice. In a radical distillation of his psychoanalytic perspective, Balint created an environment in which to examine regression in a doctor affected by the impact of a patient. Applying the theory of the "basic fault" to address forms of fault lines in communication, and of unconscious affect between doctors and their patients, the work of Balint groups allowed the unconscious dynamic of the doctor–patient interaction to emerge, as in the analytic setting. Nearly fifty years after Michael's death, groups sharing this methodology exist all over the world under the Balint name—and have also been used to develop the skills of other professional groups, including psychiatrists, nurses, the clergy, occupational therapists, and schoolteachers.

The first discussion groups for general practitioners were held at the Tavistock Clinic, where Michael Balint was a consultant psychotherapist. The original aim of these seminars was to find out what general practice was like, what was wrong with it, and to establish whether psychoanalysis, with its particular way of looking at human relationships and working with the unconscious, could be of use. The seeds for this idea began earlier, in the 1930s, when Balint first gathered together some general practitioners to try to study the psychotherapeutics in their practice. He wrote:

> I started the seminar with a series of lectures, which I know now are quite useless ... However, the political situation deteriorated further; we were ordered to notify the police of every one of our meetings, with the result that a plainclothes policeman attended each of them, taking copious notes of everything that we said. Yet the amusing outcome was that the detective always used the group to consult about himself or his family.

> (M. Balint, quoted in Stewart, 1996, p. 2)

In essence, the format that Michael and Enid Balint developed for their groups some sixty years ago remains the same today. Balint described the new field in his most influential book, *The Doctor, his Patient and the Illness* (1957). Eight to twelve general practitioners, with one or two leaders who were psychoanalysts, would meet once a week for two hours, for a minimum of two years. The group leader interviewed potential participants beforehand. For this, Balint favoured a semi-structured interview that invited the doctor to examine, perhaps for the first time, why he or she had become a doctor, and why their particular specialty or set of medical interests had been chosen. The initial interview invited the doctor to consider which types of clinical work or patients they liked and disliked treating. It became apparent through this process that the doctor's specific predilections in clinical practice were inevitably rooted in their own character and personal history. Starting to think in this way during the "Mutual Selection Interview" was itself an experiential introduction to how the Balint group worked.

Here, Balint was expressing his idea that each was interviewing the other, and that both could decide whether to accept or reject working together—the usual hierarchy thus being flattened. In particular, the value placed on the element of mutuality—that each participant had particular forms of knowledge—was established from the beginning. This was a very different atmosphere from the usual teaching position and presented a shift from the usual method of imparting medical pedagogy, which up until then invariably took the form of the master teaching the pupil.

The groups did not offer personal therapy, but there was an expectation that greater self-awareness would develop as a result of attending a Balint group over a period of time. It is important to note that, as discussions were firmly focused on the doctor–patient relationship— above all on its implications for the doctor in their stuckness, and in their difficulty in understanding the clinical encounter—the format of these groups was quite different from the usual supervision of clinical material in a group setting. As Marie Campkin (1986, p. 100) described: "Discomfort or distress in the doctor are not ignored but are worked through in the context of the needs and problems of the patient rather than of the doctor." The standard rules for small working groups applied: confidentiality, honesty, ownership, and respect for other group members. It is important to stress that the work was intended to be radically different from supervision of clinical material in a group. The supervisory type of learning is a well-known form of passing on knowledge from the teacher to the doctor, very different from a mutual system of developing understanding together. Within the Balint group, by contrast, no single person has privileged access to ideas. Although the psychoanalyst has particular knowledge about human relationships and the unconscious, the general practitioner has their own field of psychosomatic knowledge and experience.

Each session allows time for one or two new clinical presentations, as well as a follow-up of previous cases. A case history from one of the doctors might focus on their concern for a patient, on their inability to understand a clinical interaction, or on a sense of simply feeling stuck, and discussion would then be opened to the group. Matters of "fact" might need to be outlined, but only those that have a bearing on the doctor–patient relationship are deemed relevant. The group members are encouraged to free associate to the clinical material. This means that not only relevant thoughts and feelings are given an opportunity to be heard, but also seemingly irrelevant ones. The main field of clinical interest within the Balint group is the doctor's countertransference in relation to their patient. From this stems the Balints' idea that if the doctor is to develop more skills in terms of their clinical relationships with patients, they need to have a significant, thorough—albeit limited—change in their unconscious process. In practice, this can be difficult to achieve, and the group inevitably sways towards a more comfortable and passive position of wanting the leader to impart theory, or towards trying to offer the doctor personal therapy within the group context. Both of these positions are a form of group resistance to the crucial problem of the doctor–patient relationship. It is often difficult to realise when this is taking place, or to recognise the measure of psychic danger being unfolded away from the patient and into the group process. It can also be tempting to give in to the group's pressure at these moments, but when this happens it is always at the cost of attending to the doctor–patient relationship. At times, it can seem as if this relationship, together with the phantasies that are aroused, are the last things that should be discussed. This is of central importance when there seems to be a pull to "do something" other than be in the presence of the material, rather than to think through and feel it. At such times, the strength of the desire to move away from the free-associative centre may be a measure of psychic danger unfolding from the patient and being unconsciously projected, in some form, onto the presenting doctor, and then into the group process.

It is important to underline that this format is considerably different from supervision of clinical material in a group setting. I am reiterating this as it is common to hear about supervision groups,—particularly with psychiatrists, being called Balint groups when they in fact operate by just supervising the clinical case presented. The Balint group differs by specifically concentrating on the problem the psychiatrist has with his or her patient, based on specifically evoking and understanding the countertransference. Balint work is not all about teachers and the taught, nor is it about supervision. In the context of the Balint group, both of these positions can become manifestations of resistance to the unconscious impact of the clinical material. The purpose of the group is to improve the doctor's understanding of the patient's problems rather than to immediately find a solution. Inevitably, this increased knowledge is worked out in the group's relationship with the doctor who is bringing a problem in their work with the patient. Questions and advice are discouraged, but participants are encouraged to speculate and give free rein to their phantasies in order to see what they imagine is being expressed in the doctor–patient relationship. Often the presenting doctor, quite able to respond with clarity and humanity to other cases, is unable to achieve a sufficient distance from a case that has become emotionally difficult for them.

It is taken as axiomatic that knowledge of the patient and the clinical relationship resides in the mind of the presenting doctor, rather than existing in the case notes. The doctors are discouraged from reading out their clinical notes, as they need to discover what they authentically know of the interaction with their patient from within the presentation of their memory. In the telling of the clinical case, more associations to the material invariably come to mind. Vaguely remembered associations are also of interest, as they are in psychoanalysis. A doctor's colleagues can give their own thoughts in order to further develop and extend the capacity for feeling and thinking about the clinical material. Moreover, it was also accepted that second thoughts can have a value, implying a furtherance of thinking and understanding. The group tolerates the absence of a consistent story, and any muddle is instead valued and made use of. The basic understanding of this is that human beings—doctors and patients—unconsciously defend themselves from certain thoughts and ideas, and that the emergence of omissions and falsifications can lead to more understanding. Hunches, phantasies, and feelings expressed without embarrassment, in a very ordinary way, can lead to the group making psychodynamic sense of clinical material. This methodology has remained unchanged since its inception.

The observation of changes, however minute, in the doctor–patient relationship, and, in particular, in the doctor's feelings about their patient, is at the centre of this work. In 1961, the Balints published the book *Psychotherapeutic Techniques in Medicine*. Its statement was that what the patient thinks about their illness is less important than what the patient feels in the present moment, in the room with the doctor. To understand the patient, the doctor needs to listen to what they do not understand, and to be able to identify in that dyadic process. The doctor must first identify with their patient, then withdraw from that identification and become an objective professional observer again. Thus, the process of identification has a biphasic structure. This double exposure to the clinical atmosphere considerably helps orientate the doctor even when the psychic terrain is complex or seems impossible.

Six minutes for the patient

In 1966, a group of ten doctors and the two Balints met at University College Hospital (UCH), London, and worked together for five years, with the group ending a year after Michael Balint's death in 1970. The ensuing book, *Six Minutes for the Patient* (E. Balint & J. S. Solomon, 1973), described the idea of long interviews with patients in order to go deeper into what was distressing. The move to see the patient for an extended session was, in a way, mimetic of a psychoanalytic session's longer timespan of fifty minutes, as well as a response to a felt need to spend more clinical time exploring and unravelling the psychology and history of the clinical picture.

The technique that arose from the particular group at UCH was called "the flash"—a moment of apparent mutual understanding between doctor and patient, communicated by the former to the latter. This was not an understanding about the patient's past that the doctor was aware of, but something in their current life that was reflected in the relationship with the doctor for a brief time. It was an experiment that became too entrancing, however, containing as it did a sort of omnipotent magic. One problem was that the long psychodynamic interview was a foreign body in the doctors' normal routines, even if some of the participants did desire to be analysts and psychotherapists (Balint famously quipped that, however worthy it was that the individual Balint doctor was interested in training as a psychoanalyst, this would mean a loss of talent to general practice).

In time, it was discovered that what was paramount were the changes and adjustments to the doctor's feelings about the patient, and vice versa—changes that were not necessarily communicated at the time. If the doctor had a sense of understanding their patient at a particular consultation, then at a subsequent meeting there would be a change in doctor's state of mind. They would be more receptive, perhaps, more knowing, more aware, and less negative, angry, confused, or hostile towards the patient. Even with nothing being said, a new atmosphere (the *arglos* state) could develop, which the patient could unconsciously accept, making possible a new direction for the doctor–patient relationship that was more creative for both of them. The patient might perhaps experience an atmosphere of being enjoyed by the doctor, who, for a change, was not seen to be reaching for the prescription pad as soon as the patient entered in order to bring about their rapid departure. The patient felt welcomed despite the burdens being brought.

This process involves the development of a clinical relationship over time. It is far more than just dealing with the particular medical problem, as, in addition, it offers the doctor a profound role in the imaginative perception of the patient's unconscious expectations, which are based on the latter's personal history. It allows the patient to move towards a more creative—and, ultimately, more real—form of object relationship with the world. The finding of an object that understands can suggest the rediscovery of a type of good object that had been "lost", but it can also imply the development and establishment of a good object relationship with the other (the doctor, in their role as a primal figure) for the first time in the patient's life. By this, I mean the unexpected discovery by a patient suffering from early trauma that there may be someone with concern for their welfare, and that they are not so alone in the world.

This is particularly relevant when the patient's need to display symptoms can be a psychosomatic cipher for communicating that "something is wrong" at a deep psychological level. The hearing, understanding doctor, in their role as a new type of receptive object, meets the patient in a fresh light. At the commencement of this type of new beginning it is especially important to realise that there is no need to disturb the patient by telling them that they may be starting to have, perhaps for the first time, an existential hope in the world. Instead, the patient and doctor are allowed to feel freely and quietly pleased to be looking forward to the next meeting. In heart-sink cases, this clinical development can be an extraordinary discovery. The impossible patient, unconsciously representing their problematic childhood through their symptoms and character, can now start to be perceived in a more benign and quiet state. This is not the same as an analysis, but it can provide a shaft of light that allows the clinical dyad to function together in an atmosphere of concern. It can be thought of as a beginning that the patient takes away, and which they may, or may not, be unconsciously able to use. This is a profound reason for the patient's doctor to remain as a specific, stable object that can be re-found again and again. The specificity and reliability of the particular doctor, in opposition to the factory mentality that any doctor on duty will suffice, plays a profound role in the patient having a new and continuing realisation that they are worthy of being looked after.

As previously stated, the work of the group is not about a supervision that allows free play of the clinical material in order to understand the patient; the entirety of the work is about understanding the unconscious relationship of the doctor and patient from the vicissitudes of the countertransference of the doctor. The obvious pitfall is that the therapist, as leader, may concentrate more on the individual or group dynamics of what is under discussion, and thus unwittingly move away from the specific Balint model of the relationship. This is made more likely by the fact that the Balint method may superficially resemble other psychodynamic modes of work with colleagues. On the contrary, however, being much more akin to enabling a psychoanalytic atmosphere in which free associations can be developed and understood within the group—specifically in relation to what can be understood through the prism of countertransference—the Balint method provides a very different model from all other types of supervision. The work is not necessarily about understanding the clinical material of the patient. Rather, the centre of the clinical gaze is on the countertransference of the doctor—on what their problem or resistance to being able to know, understand, and work with the patient is. The other doctors in the group invariably have a flexibility of thought and affect about the case presented, as does the presenter when listening to other presentations. And so it is the presenting doctor's unconscious resistance that is the core of the listening process in the Balint group, and this is much more defined in focus than a general psychodynamic supervision. This is the reason for rejecting the idea that any psychotherapist or psychoanalyst can run a Balint group, as running these groups requires induction to the methodology and specificity of their focus.

The characters and personal histories of the group members form crucial elements on which the clinical work invariably depends. Learning in this field thus often requires a considerable shift in a doctor's character. If, for instance, a similar structural difficulty is repeatedly brought by one of the doctors to the group, without any movement or development, this might be an indication that the doctor would benefit from seeking a private solution somewhere separately, perhaps undergoing their own analysis. However, the movements that occur in the group usually enable subtle character shifts in the doctor to occur quietly and concomitantly with a greater understanding of the clinical material.

The countertransference

I now want to examine in more detail what goes on in the Balint group. There are three levels of countertransference reaction to be discerned:

- the relationship between doctor and patient;
- the relationship between doctor and group leader;
- the relationship between doctor and other group members.

The group leader unconsciously functions as a superego, representing the standards and knowledge ideally being aimed for. When a doctor is interviewing a patient it becomes common that the group leader is in the doctor's mind. Sometimes the clinical interview is then conducted in order to show that the group leader is wrong, or is wonderful, or that the doctor has learnt their lessons. Similar attitudes may permeate the group, but such material, whilst often present, should only be sparingly touched upon, over-emphasis moving the direction of the work towards group psychotherapy.

It can be helpful to perceive the group of doctors as rivalrous siblings, reflecting the dynamics of Freud's primal horde (Freud, 1912–1913, p. 141). Occasionally, the group can quickly move away from the psychodynamic centre of the clinical picture in an unconscious attempt to neutralise their leader. It is the leader's task to liberate the group and, when members become stuck in their deliberations, to voice criticism in a constructive, unaggressive manner. Within the group, sheer aggression is only destructive hatred and, as such, is useless, in the same way that its opposite, sugar-coated idealisation—suggesting that all is wonderful—is also useless. The emotional balance can be hard to achieve, takes time to develop, and may happen in a very piecemeal way—yet it must be maintained. If there are hesitations or long silences, or if the group has been acting too kindly, then the leader can speak about the atmosphere, relating back to some hidden aspect of the clinical problem. The leader is also there to stop one member being repeatedly interrogated. The presenter can sometimes be bombarded with questions as if they have all the answers. Making the doctor–patient dyad the central focus is an unusual medical innovation more akin to the techniques of psychoanalysis. It is a mode of work that brings with it states of resistance which must be faced and understood, meaning that groups can at times be hypercritical, bland, indifferent, bored, or uncooperative—all as resistances to deepening the understanding of the clinical material. All of these dynamics require careful and minimal intervention from the group leader, who needs to listen to the clinical presentation together with the associations coming from the members of the group. The holding function of the leader requires no intervention unless the group is ignoring an important direction. Here it is crucially important for the leader to be able to hear and feel unconscious resonances in the work, and to sense the resistances in the group, as well as to find the interpretative sentence that may allow the work to deepen and progress.

The group leader will invariably have gained from having had the experience of previously attending a Balint group themselves. A leader without such personal experience would need to attend a Balint leaders' workshop on an ongoing and regular basis in order to learn the new methodology. Such workshops, together with a working understanding of individual and group psychodynamics, are of great use. Psychoanalysts and well-trained psychoanalytic psychotherapists, as well as talented general practitioners who have initially co-led in a Balint group, can offer leadership. If a leader has not been apprenticed in a Balint group it is difficult to imagine how they might lead one. In such situations the individual usually misunderstands their role as being based on a leader in normal group psychotherapy. This may be of some interest, but the group becomes skewed into providing case material for dynamic supervision. This is not the Balint model, which insists on making the doctor–patient dyad the centre of focus.

As the Balint methodology has unfolded and developed over the years it has been taken up with enthusiasm throughout Europe and the US as a way for young doctors to deepen the psychological component and practice of their clinical work. It has similarly been applied to develop the training of junior psychiatrists. Nonetheless, the name "Balint" is often misused as a catch-all category for supervision or the discussion of clinical work that has nothing to do with this model of thought. A patient's illness or "stuckness" can be better examined, and have its grip more easily loosened, by the doctor who can find change in themselves, a position at the furthest remove from—and designed to prevent—the unconscious projections of a doctor onto a so-called "impossible" patient.

Psychosomatics and early life

Psychosomatics is a very interesting arena to examine within the Balint group, as the illness brought by the patient can show the development of a gap between the body and the mind that contains lost affect. In psychosomatic presentations, often the body-ego has taken the psychic burden for things that the patient feels should not be thought and felt in the mind, or spoken about. For patients who are overflowing with such intensities, it becomes a necessity to unconsciously transfer them to the body and into a state of physical illness. As how the patient may experience and feel about their illness is perceived by the doctor as irrelevant, usually only the problem with and in the body is examined. Often, however, the lost affects can be located in some aspect of the transference with the doctor. During a clinical presentation, a doctor's ability to notice that affect and thought are being left out—and that there is a consistent dwelling on the ailments of the body, and on medication—can lead to an awareness of an absence, or that affects are being projected onto them. The doctor can often recognise these lost affects, coming from the patient, through a consideration of their own feeling state in the clinical encounter. Similarly, such analytical methodology can examine the world of the unhappy and frightened child that might be located somewhere within the adult patient as an illness, but which can often be projected onto a spouse, or child, or doctor. Patients that appear to be in charge of the clinical encounter can often be a source of great upset to the doctor, who feels they are only being used as a cipher to obtain drugs or letters of support to government agencies. Discovering such emotions is a step towards a deeper understanding of how the doctor is being made use of, however, together with how the dynamic resonates both with the patient's expectations of relationships generally, and with their early history. Often, with thought, one can rediscover the ordinariness and prosaic character in the psychic issue. In other words, a finding of a piece of the history or affect that, when articulated, becomes something that is obvious to both doctor and patient, and something which can facilitate clinical movement.

Balint thought of this type of work as research. The ability to make and test a hypothesis with the follow-up to the case, at the next appointment for instance, is of importance to the development of the doctor's capacity to think. Part of the research in examining hypotheses is what might develop for the patient within their family life. This can be a long process, as the patient may not reappear for another consultation for a considerable time. The work is often attended to at the patient's pace. Whilst this is similar to the analytic model (that it is unwise to make an interpretation until one thinks that the patient is in a state of mind to receive it), nonetheless there is no demand that the patient attends several sessions each week. The family doctor, however, does sometimes have, usually in contrast to psychoanalysis, the potential for a heightened emotional understanding in being able to see the patient in the environment of their own home, with its kitchen and its bedrooms. The home space can be profoundly evocative in understanding the clinical background.

Development in the doctor attending the Balint group can be observed in the changes in the way they talk about clinical work and relate to their group colleagues. The Balint methodology is a melding of the psychic and somatic, with the potential to understand the impact of the patient's early environment on their character and on their forms of physical and mental illnesses. A possibility that a doctor continues to provide care for a baby through the life cycle—through childhood and into adulthood—can enable a deep psychosocial understanding of the patient within the context of family life. This profound knowledge can be transformative for clinical work, but requires the long-term dyadic link between doctors and patients to be respected. This is a very different medicine to that which is becoming the norm, modelled on factory production, including such demands as that patients see the next available doctor. Such an impoverished understanding of medical care is an attack on the relevance and vitality not only of essential historical knowledge but, more deeply, of the doctor's functioning in the life and family setting of the patient.

Doctors and psychoanalysts: the transference and the countertransference

The model of the Balint group creates and makes use of a reciprocal relationship between the professionals taking part. It is an unusual model, in that learning is non-hierarchical and a two-way process. The doctors and the psychoanalyst learn from the clinical material in the presentation, and from their associations and interactions, in a way that is similar and mindful of the analytic dyad. The conversations between the medical practitioners and the psychoanalyst are ones involving respect for each other's knowledge. The analyst in the Balint group does not need to have had a medical training. Enid Balint was awarded an honorary membership of the Royal College of General Practitioners for her work with the profession.

What an analyst brings to such a group is a particular form of listening to clinical material—a form of "being in the experience" with what is being discussed. This is necessarily very different from the position first taken by the doctors attending, who bring a medical case formulation, with a differential diagnosis and often a treatment plan, in the usual inductive way they have been trained to think. The case is brought as a clinical problem in which something has gone wrong, the presenting doctor feeling out of their depth. The patient may have ignored the doctor's advice, or it has been unhelpful, and the doctor might foster a private belief that the patient is somehow being impossible. This new engagement with problems of the "heart", translated as emotion, is the beginning of a realisation of a new strand in medical understanding and concern—even of medical ethics. The doctor, who works with a method of communication that usually—one could say unconsciously—functions, now finds from the perspective of a particular doctor–patient dyad that it fails him. The presenting doctor's colleagues in the group often have less or no difficulty evaluating the clinical picture in a new light, and the doctor is forced to realise that the character and unconscious emotional life of their patient is a particular problem for themselves, as doctor. Realisation that the problem resides in the area of the doctor's own private feelings and phantasies becomes the royal road to a greater clinical understanding, which in time may have an effect on their own character—something often sensed unconsciously by their patient. A patient's emotional associations and identifications can often be projected onto an other, the doctor finding themselves full of affect that appears to be ego dystonic, experiencing feelings and perhaps even thoughts that are felt to be strange—different from how they usually see and feel about the world and themselves. Sometimes this is due to the force of some particular psychic vulnerability in the doctor themselves, because of the history of their own family life. If the doctor can bear to acknowledge and consciously engage with such emotive strands, this countertransference material becomes a psychological element in the mind of the doctor that can lead to an improved clinical understanding of the emotional difficulties of the patient.

The doctor ideally comes to realise that there is no such thing as a clinical medicine that is not entangled with the particularities, peculiarities, and individuality of the doctor practising their medical work—with their likes and dislikes, prejudices, pleasures, and hatreds, feelings that usually dwell beneath the contents of a reported clinical encounter, repressed beneath professional demeanour. Almost repressed, that is, as the doctor usually has a private, fleeting thought, for example: "This patient is always interesting; I look forward to meeting her", or, "That one always disturbs me." Such psychology, especially concerning the self, is invariably not taught in medical school, nor is it regarded as being a useful part of the clinical picture. It is not like the science of pulse-taking, or reading an electrocardiogram or X-ray. It is more likely to be regarded as scatological, sexual, irrelevant, and not particularly worthy of being considered part of "proper" medicine. This brings us back to psychoanalysis, which today is similarly regarded as clinically irrelevant to medicine. Character is usually not thought to be part of the medical picture, and it may not need to be until the doctor finds there is a problem or a difficulty understanding in the clinical encounter. With a patient that the doctor finds almost impossible to understand, or even tolerate, they are forced to admit their own difficulties being creative in their usual way in their work with patients. This is often regarded as a clash of personality, and this alone should elicit curiosity rather than being considered to be unrelated to the clinical problem. I am not describing a lack of medical talent in the doctor, nor a lacuna in medical knowledge, but rather that a particular doctor is unable to make good clinical use of themselves, with a particular patient. Interaction between the characters involved in a clinical encounter then requires a deepened understanding—something not necessarily readily available following the rigours of a general medical education, nor even specialisation, other than through the subject of psychoanalysis. These characters are the representations of the other, which each party unconsciously perceives in the encounter. In a somewhat obvious way, the doctor can often readily perceive themselves being in the role of a father—either a new, wise one who might be helpful, or perhaps the re-embodiment of an original father perceived as difficult, unhelpful, or even dangerous. One can consider the same imaginative circuit in terms of the maternal object, or similarly the sibling relationship, these characters being available for both the patient and their doctor to inhabit and enact. The same dynamics can be thought about in terms of the sexuality of such representation. This can be of particular interest as the clinical encounter is often a presentation of part of the body, requiring the doctor to be able to deal with the physical aspect of their patient, as well as enlarging their understanding of the psychological meaning of the part of the body being offered to them. The utility of such awareness in the moment of the consultation is that something of primitive and early relationships can emerge in that setting—the child in the adult being revealed, seemingly hindering the doctor's work, or, more interestingly, providing clues to the early development of their patient's unconscious relationships. At times, this early history can have a profound bearing on why the patient presents, as well as having an impact on the types of symptoms they are dealing with in their body.

The psychoanalyst in the analytic dyad, knowing something more of their own character and passions from their personal analysis, can occupy a more neutral and observing position towards the developing relationship. Being sensitive to the unconscious—both their own and that of the analysand—enables the analyst in their freely associative state to be more in touch with the age-old analytic question of "who is doing what, to whom, and why". This leads to the possibility of allowing more thought and less action. Reflective thought, even in the presence of emotional disturbance, can enable greater creative possibility with the patient than a thoughtless knee-jerk reaction, wishing to quickly escape the tension in the consulting room. The analyst is neither too friendly nor too distant, but is present to think and be thoughtful back, as initially described and recommended by Freud: "The doctor should be opaque to his patients and, like a mirror, should show them nothing but what is shown to him" (1912e, p. 118). If such neutrality is not possible, the doctor should be at least free to notice the position they are occupying in the patient's narrative—the "transference"—as well as the private feelings being agitated in the clinical encounter. The analyst, responding as a human being, does not thrust their personality onto the patient. There is no demand that the particular medicine—analytic insight—must be taken. The patient's ability to perceive reality varies at different times. This is certainly truer when a patient, facing a crisis, visits their doctor. At such times, a medical crisis may well be found to be a somatic expression of very tense emotions. For instance, it is highly likely that some patients do not suffer heart attacks out of the blue; rather, they can be a serious somatic counterpoint to what the heart is unable to bear emotionally. The history-taking of what was happening in the patient's life and imagination prior to the onset of the illness is often very instructive in understanding what initially appears to be only a malady in the body. Was there a profound emotional rupture that the heart was unable to bear? Such an actuality—in addition to the damage inflicted on the heart muscle itself, and its subsequently increased vulnerability—may have long-term implications for the likelihood of another attack.

Different patients see us differently and we are seen in as many ways as we have patients. Doctors can sometimes have an awareness of this, but this can be obscured by being over-concerned with the presentation of one part of the patient's body—the part offered to the doctor to be seen. There is no such thing as the body of a patient, however, that is separate from their mind—a patient cannot bring only their body to the doctor or analyst. Unfortunately, many medical specialists assess the patient in terms of an isolated pathology, such that the reality of a whole person as patient can go unnoticed.

A very important Arab dignitary, in London for his regular medical visit, was seated on a throne in the centre of his large hotel suite, surrounded by his specialists from Harley Street. The cardiologist, urologist, and chest physician were all in attendance, but felt powerless in treating his complaint of an intense ache on one side of his head. None of the distinguished specialist physicians had the right expertise to examine his ear, except perhaps the less illustrious general practitioner, who was also present. Despite feeling out of his depth, it was left to him to examine the prince, in full view of the roomful of very senior but impotent doctors. As he began to put the otoscope towards his patient's ear he was leant on by an over-vigilant bodyguard, worried that his charge might be stabbed. Nonetheless, he persisted enough in the examination to remove a large solid wax ball impacted in the ear. The prince felt his ear pop, the pain left at once, and hearing was immediately restored. This example demonstrates the limitations of specialised medicine as well as a doctor's anxiety and fear in the presence of a powerful patient and senior professionals. Whole-person medicine, as practised by the competent general practitioner, can be essential, with much greater success than a specialist who examines a part-body complaint, and can often render only a partial solution.

The analyst may be perceived as a cold, rigid person by one patient, and a warmer one by another, each perceived analyst perhaps containing parental fragments of expectation and desire. Similarly, our age varies according to the patient's imagination. This is also true in general practice. The analyst's perception of the patient is made up of a substratum of clinical data that is linked to the patient's early life; the family constellation; how early loss and illness was dealt with within the family; aspects of feeling and of being either loved or abandoned, hated, or abused; and whether these events and their feelings took place in the context of a parental couple or a single parent, all of which is etched onto the personality and a person's expectations of an imagined future. This early life, unconsciously perceived, makes itself available through its projection onto the important imagined character of the analyst—or the medical doctor. There is an unconscious capacity for the doctor to play deep unconscious roles, and this can often be as a healer—one who makes the hurt better. However, it is also possible for negative aspects of a patient's mental life to be superimposed on, or to be active beneath, the clinical work—expectations projected onto the future and derived from past experiences, both real and imagined. And so a patient's inexplicable rage with their doctor may be an emotional shard that has arisen from the past, uneasily laying itself on top of the present interaction. The analyst knows well enough that it may not be themselves per se that the analysand is experiencing but rather, regressed to the child, the unconscious projection onto them of the parent, perhaps. The doctor needs to evaluate if they have really done something wrong, or whether they just feel that they have, in which case the doctor is "in role" in the patient's history. Awareness of this process is a central method of clinical evidence in the Balint group, on a par with measuring the pulse or electrolyte balance in medical practice.

By gathering the impressions of psychosomatic material through sensing what seems to be happening in the relationship, the doctor is in a stronger clinical position to evaluate the physical illness in the context of the patient's emotive relational environment. Some of the projections onto the doctor can then start to be understood, rather than reacted against. It is important to note the ambiguity of who does the understanding here. It is possible that the understanding the doctor can have about their patient can be talked about with them, leading to maturation, and emotional, and even physical improvement. It can at least help to create a better clinical atmosphere for doing further medical work. But it may also be sufficient—or may be the only possibility at that moment—that the knowledge and understanding stays inside the doctor. At least the doctor may not then be at their wits' end in not comprehending the encounter, making them better able to understand and work out, over time, a more appropriate emotional contact with their patient. The impetus for the doctor to rid themselves of their impossible patient will almost certainly have receded. In the analytic model this sort of internal awareness is equivalent to the timing of an interpretation. Just because the analyst has perceived something that may be meaningful, and that might have value in being communicated, does not mean it is the right time for it to be given to the patient to try swallowing and digesting it. Both analyst and doctor may need to wait for an opportunity to speak. In general practice such a slow burn in the unfolding of the clinical knowledge of the patient, often within the context of their family, is normal. The patient continues to attend the surgery for whatever reason and gradually their doctor builds up a complex understanding of them and their family life over many years. It used to be common that a doctor would know a family through three generations of its life. The doctor would be immersed in family matters as an "outside insider", a specialist in knowing the family in a clinical way. This good model of the family doctor is sadly being wiped out by the exiguousness of financial systems that dictate that the next doctor should see the next patient, rather than the embedded doctor. We are informed that this is cheaper and more efficient medicine, but it is in fact a much costlier model, as the underlying and often subtle knowledge of the patient and their family history is being wiped out. Family medicine, shorn of its historical and generational context, is being replaced with an industrial and mechanistic medicine that values only the isolated time of the medical event, with another unfamiliar doctor.

Let us return to the clinical dyad, where there is further movement to consider. The doctor who is always stirred by an enraged patient to defend themselves, or to retaliate, may, with an understanding of what we have been discussing, be suddenly interested in their patient in new ways. Now not needing to defend themselves, from what had seemed to be the patient's capricious emotions, the doctor can become a more solid base for their patient. It may well be that in the case of more regressed patients there is a greater necessity for the doctor to be a firm, non-retaliatory, and solid figure who begins to hold the patient in their emotional struggles without having to be doctor, mother, father, and agonist or antagonist. In other words, there might be more need for the doctor to just be there as a friendly substrate. This in itself may be unusual and helpful.

To return now to Freud's idea of the analyst as mirror, and to his recommendation that "the doctor should be opaque to his patients ... [showing] them nothing but what is shown to him" (Freud, 1912e, p. 118). If this methodology is maintained too rigidly, however, an analyst might repeat some of the patient's traumas, the consequences of which had brought the patient to analysis. For instance, if the parents were also opaque in that manner, the analyst would only be repeating a sense of distant trauma. Enid Balint brings an interesting twist to these ideas in her remarks on Freud's metaphor about the "mirror" and the "receiver":

> More than the patient, it is the analyst who has difficulties in adhering to the mirror model. When we are tired and not on our guard, we may find ourselves paying less attention to the association of ideas, which is hard work, and instead discover that we are listening to a description of events in the patient's life which we might like to respond to in a friendly way. If we do this, we show the kind of people we are: we deviate from the mirror model; but more often than the patient, I think it is we who wish to deviate from the model.

> (E. Balint, 1968, p. 59)

She continues with the thought that, for some patients, when the analyst is friendlier or more sympathetic, having deviated from the distanced model, the part of them that is well may show satisfaction or gratification, but the part of them that is ill may feel alienated, ignored, and unhelped. In this sense the analytic distance is that creative tool that can enable the analyst to just be there, a kind of substrate—as described by Michael Balint (1959, p. 95), and as noted earlier.

For patients who are more seriously ill, being a substrate for them can be a more effective clinical position, as it means that the analyst is not just perceived or transferentially cast as a particular character or set of affects that the patient continues to have difficulty understanding or dealing with. At times the analyst's words may be experienced as impingements or distortions, and often seen as signs of hostility or seduction. Nonetheless, such feelings in the patient of the analyst's apparent antagonism can also reveal a deep chasm of pain and hurt residing in some area of their shrouded history. These matters need to be reflected on and remembered, and a structure provided to try to understand the heightened emotional relating taking place in the encounter (whilst not offering interpretations that may only be heard as a continuation of attacks on the patient, or of them not being understood). Whilst this sort of understanding is an ideal state, when working with a regressed patient it is very often the case that the analyst has already fallen down some awful black hole—perhaps as the only way of discovering the terrible terrain lying beneath the surface material of good working relations. The analyst needs to recover through the biphasic possibilities of first identifying with the patient and then returning to their own self by disidentifying, in order to balance the clinical material with understanding, beyond the initial affect of falling into an emotional abyss. Sometimes this is the only way that a regressed patient can communicate their reality to the analyst. Furthermore, it often signifies that the patient has fallen into some deep emotional hole earlier in their upbringing, the analyst's fall being a repetition of an earlier mental event, real or imagined, resurrected in the present moment. The reasons for this occurring are often complex. It may indicate that such a way of behaving has been the only narrow possibility for emotional communication available to the patient for a long time. Yet it is also a communication of such a state of being with the other. The replay of past relations can be straightforward, in the sense that the analyst is perhaps unconsciously expected to play the role of the parent in the old regime. They can also be enacted in the opposite direction, however, so that the patient, after identifying with the parent, is doing to the other what they had felt done to them, earlier in their life. This defence enables the patient to avoid being on the receiving end again, whilst at the same time unconsciously allowing the other to feel something of what it had been like to be treated in "that way". Such clinical material often has to remain as something perplexing, and even to be continuously enacted—a form of dealing with it (badly), until, in time, and with enough repetition, understanding of the past emerges in the present.

This is a description of difficulties in the analytic encounter, but how is this relevant to general medical practice? The answer is that, very often, ill patients will unconsciously regard the doctor as a parent of their past, and it is this connection that can suddenly unleash an emotional outpouring that can seem, from the doctor's perspective, to come out of nowhere. The patient that attends with a problem with part of their body suddenly emotionally erupts with a challenge to the doctor. The essential link is that the doctor is in a privileged and intimate position in relation to the patient's body, on a par only with parents and lovers. In many ways the doctor has more such privilege than the analyst as they can enter the patient's house and bedroom as well as being in contact with parts of their body. It is a normal expectation that you "put yourself in the hands of the doctor". Such literalness suggests the primitive desire to be held, as the baby by the mother, in a "good enough way"; and so, the potential for emotional representation lies in the powerful connections of transference and their impact on mind and body. The physician's privileged position with regard to the body is paralleled by the analyst's position with regard to the conscious and unconscious mind. The doctor, finding themselves suddenly forced to defend some emotional position that seems so far away from the initial medical enquiry, can take some solace from the fact that it probably has very little to do with them personally—only with them being in a particular role for their patient. The first two of the following vignettes describe the impact of the clinical encounter on the medical practitioner in relation to a fragment from their own past that has re-emerged in the material. In these cases, we see how associations to the perhaps unprocessed thoughts of the respective doctors led, in the Balint group, to ideas of how they could help their patients, consequent to the doctors each beginning to free themselves of their own separate and private histories.

Clinical vignettes of Balint groups with general practitioners

> In this work activity of a special kind is released in the doctors, a kind of psychic activity. Liveliness: not passive acceptance. Observations: not instructions.

> (Enid Balint, 1987, p. 102)

Case 1: a complex medical problem and a ghost

A general practitioner presented a case of a forty-five-year-old woman who had attended for a single consultation with the presenting complaint of having red spots on her legs. Dr A told the group, with some pride, that she had a great deal of clinical experience in the field of dermatology. She told the group that she had become quite an expert, to the extent that she was known as the "spot doc" in her clinical practice. She thought that the diagnosis was either cellulitis or erythema nodosum. During the consultation, and with the patient in the room, Dr A phoned her former colleague, a consultant dermatologist, who recommended that the diagnosis was most likely to be cellulitis. On his recommendation, Dr A gave the patient a prescription for penicillin. However, Dr A really thought that her other diagnosis of erythema nodosum was probably more likely.

Three days later, blood tests confirmed that her suspicion was indeed correct, and she sent the patient to have an X-ray, due to concern about another possible complication called sarcoid. This X-ray did in fact show that the patient had unusual nodules in her chest. To Dr A's horror, the hospital radiographer suggested that the patient have a mediastinal biopsy, and, as this was complicated, she might even have to have a thoracotomy (a large operation to open a gap through the ribs in order to take the biopsy from inside the chest). Dr A, in some distress, rang the patient, who after arriving with spots on her legs was suddenly being invited to have a major surgical procedure. The patient reacted stoically to the direction of the investigation, however, saying that if there was something wrong then it needed to be properly examined, and telling the doctor that she had, in fact, already had the biopsy.

The doctor sent a letter to the consultant dermatologist and received a response stating that the situation was unusual because the biopsy stain did not look like a picture of sarcoid, and that the diagnosis was probably tuberculosis. Despite the fact that the case was becoming more complicated, Dr A again accepted the consultant's advice that the patient should immediately start triple therapy for tuberculosis, even though the result of further diagnostic blood cultures would not be known for several weeks. The patient then made an appointment to see Dr A and said that she was now very worried because, if this treatment was instituted, she would have to take sixteen hundred tablets over the next three months. The patient was actually feeling healthy, and was concerned that taking so many tablets might make her ill. It was this dilemma that Dr A brought to the Balint group.

Everybody in the group agreed with the notion that the treatment offered was excessive, considering that, if the patient did have tuberculosis, waiting another few weeks for the test results would not make any real difference to the treatment of her condition, as there was no open lesion that could infect others. Equally, if the diagnosis was sarcoid there was no treatment that could be offered, so either way the patient did not need urgent medication. This led the group to wonder what the doctor's problem might be in this case. When Dr A had been a student, the present consultant dermatologist was her registrar in the medical firm that she was attached to.

Since that time, and following a further placement at the hospital, she had always looked up to him.

The group wondered whether Dr A had been able to think of herself as a competent middle-aged doctor, on a par, as it were, with a consultant specialist, or whether she still considered this senior dermatologist to be "a most superior colleague". Dr A agreed that it was probably the case that she was still in awe of the older doctor, and still unconsciously taking a student role next to him. It was difficult for her to accept that the consultant—who, in her eyes, had always been good, caring, and above all conservative in his clinical practice—was actually now being perceived as rather "gung-ho" in rushing to medicate the patient. She found it very hard to approach the consultant and asked the group how she might discuss the situation with him. Some of the group, knowing this particular consultant, suggested he would have no problem in accepting the need for a second opinion. It seemed that this was the end of the case, but Dr A said she had been thinking even more about why the situation had occurred, and wanted to tell a further story. The work and atmosphere in the group had freed up an unconscious memory in the doctor, leading her to have a free association. When Dr A had been a student, the very first patient she had clerked on the ward was a dermatology case. She was working in the unit of a most eminent dermatologist, in which the present consultant was, at that time, a registrar. That first patient had presented with a mild temperature and some redness on her body but had subsequently become very ill, and the consultant had commented that the young student would need to examine the patient with great care. Rapidly, this patient became extremely ill and died, despite having been given a huge amount of steroids for an illness that had first appeared as being very minor. Dr A, then a student, had privately thought that the patient had died of a steroid overdose given by the registrar.

It now gradually became clear that what was generating anxiety in her current case was the ghost of the unconscious memory of her first clinical case—one that, she discovered, was still haunting her. Dr A could even remember the name of her first patient and, furthermore, thought that she probably still retained a copy of the original file in her office. This indicated a great anxiety and unconscious preoccupation with the idea that the present case was going to be a re-run of that awful first case, in which the "Superior Consultant", then a hospital registrar, appeared to offer a massive dose of medication to a very ill patient, who then died. There seemed to be so many points of similarity in the two cases that Dr A was very relieved to have been able to link them; and to realise that her present predicament contained the shadow of her first clinical encounter, from which she, as a young doctor, had never fully recovered.

One of the main points of this vignette is to show the power and the impact of early clinical cases on a medical student. If something goes wrong, the experience can leave a psychological scar by being left unmourned in the mind of the doctor, who is then left unconsciously awaiting its repetition. The alternative is to work through the painful event in a different way. In this case, Dr A was most grateful to be reminded that she was no longer a medical student and could actually speak "doctor-to-doctor" with the consultant. In reality, he understood far better than she had imagined when thinking of him as the "consultant on high" who she had looked up to as a young student. There was evidence that she had dealt with her anxiety about her first clinical case by utilising the state of an idealisation of the senior doctor. Yet unconsciously, beneath this attitude, she had been very concerned by the death of the patient. It is unknowable whether the dying patient was treated properly or was over-medicated. Perhaps the young Dr A had never been able to reach an opinion, leaving instead an oscillation between cause and effect, and a degree of vulnerability in herself. Now Dr A could be more thoughtful and could question the urgent desire to provide medication in her present case. She was also much more aware of her clinical concerns for her patient—concerns which had unconsciously enabled an ancient and upsetting case from the past to re-emerge. Clinically, Dr A was now back in charge of the illness of her patient and felt a renewed sense of confidence about how to proceed.

As doctors, most of us have our early cases and case observations—and the impacts of various horrors from medical practice—still inside us, so to speak. Medical students are invariably young and often have less experience of life, especially of the minutiae of death. (Of course, this is not always the case, as many individuals are unconsciously brought into the profession due to early experiences of illness and mortality. The powerlessness of the child's position becomes galvanised as a need both to know and to heal others later in life.) Early medical cases, when a young doctor has no structure to locate, let alone contain, the impact of death—and of a psychic wound often perceived as powerlessness—can become a piece of unresolved mourning, even more so if it impinges on childhood traumata. The experience becomes buried soon enough, but the doctor may have a vague awareness that certain medical subjects are off limits. Sometimes, as in this instance, the early cases return, haunting their clinical work.

Case 2: the impact of dying

Dr B presented clinical material about a family situation that, privately, she found to be very upsetting. She believed that her own feelings had been interfering with her usual clinical practice, which was why she desired to present the case. An elderly man, who had been her patient for many years, had been diagnosed with a brain tumour and was gradually dying. Despite physical deterioration, the patient was nonetheless mentally alert and was being nursed at home. The doctor had been visiting every week and discovered that the usually ebullient man, who shared her interest in sport, had "turned his face to the wall", longing to die. The patient's wife seemed more concerned with her husband's bedroom being moved to the ground-floor living room, and had just arranged for the carpets to be cleaned. When the doctor arrived she was informed that as the carpets were still damp she needed to remove her shoes, in case dog excrement was brought into the house. The doctor, surprised at this beginning to the visit, did as instructed.

Dr B felt that the distant atmosphere in her patient's home was due to his rather cold wife, who now informed her that her husband could no longer speak. This was despite the fact that the doctor had recently been having very meaningful discussions with the patient. Dr B sensed that the wife wanted her husband dead as his state of illness interfered with her obsessional need for cleanliness and tidiness in their home. It was as if she wanted both her husband and the doctor to disappear because they were both bringing some sort of disturbing mess into the usually ordered house. Dr B found herself feeling very angry towards the wife, especially as she made it clear that she wanted her husband to be nursed away from the house that had been his home for so long. She recognised that the way a family deals with death is their moral right, but she felt very distressed that the kind old man she knew as her patient was being ignored and badly treated at the end of his life. Dr B said that the man had toiled all his life to make enough money for the family, and that after providing so much he did not deserve to be treated with such contempt.

The doctor found the Balint group to be a safe place to express her private feelings of rage. The patient had in fact been in a private hospital for diagnosis but, after five weeks, the health insurer, realising that the initial diagnostic task had been achieved, declined to pay anything further other than for nursing care on the acute ward. The doctor had phantasised about punishing the wife by increasing the amount of home nursing, so as to keep the husband in the house. On discussion with the other group members, she knew that this was not her moral right. The other doctors felt that the possibilities of home nursing were not necessarily the best clinical solution. In fact, they raised the possibility that the real issue of the patient's imminent death was being avoided. Dr B accepted this, realising that this idea also included her pain from losing a patient who she had admired and enjoyed treating over the years. It was very painful for the doctor to discuss this with her patient, even though she had spoken about dying and death to many of her patients over the years. She had even spoken about such matters when other colleagues had presented such difficulties themselves within the group.

Two weeks later, the doctor brought a follow-up of the case: the patient had now been placed in a hospice. Dr B's idea was to introduce a new regime that was focused on helping her patient towards death, but she had also thought that the family needed respite. Seemingly as a result of the move, the patient was no longer facing the wall and was more alive within himself. It was unclear whether the hospice could continue to keep the patient, his death no longer imminent, but it was also clear that the wife, although conversing again with her husband, did not want him to return home. Surprisingly, the doctor continued to voice her contempt for the wife even more vigorously. The group could not understand Dr B's feelings: the clinical situation was improving, the patient was in good hands, work on dying was being approached by the hospice team—and yet ...!

Spontaneously, Dr B then told the group that she now knew why she was finding the case so difficult. The group suddenly found itself in the realms of the personal—a very difficult place to be, as the focus of the group is always the doctor–patient relationship. However, Dr B's self-exploration needed to continue. She had been reminded that, several years before, a good friend of hers had died and she knew that her feelings for the patient had reawakened these earlier memories. Her feelings were particularly exacerbated because her friend's husband had been similarly obsessed with cleanliness, and he too had detested the mess of his wife's dying and had ignored his wife, leading her to wish for her own death. Whilst not the family doctor, Dr B had eventually spoken to the husband because of her concern about her friend's medical deterioration. Dr B had suggested that she be nursed in a hospice rather than within the family. Since then, her relations with the husband had been very strained, and she felt very unforgiving of his distance during the last few weeks of her friend's life.

The current clinical picture and the identification from years before was a painful matter for the doctor. Her feelings for the patient's wife were clearly suffused with hostile feelings towards her dead friend's husband. An aspect of the doctor's personal life had been unravelled by the case, and, in remaining under her skin, had prevented her usual careful and projection-free approach to clinical work. Within the context of a containing group of colleagues, she felt safe enough to reveal an aspect of her work and private life—something that she initially found humiliating, being unable to discriminate between her private past and the clinical present. The narration of the historical template released Dr B from casting projections from her own past onto her patient. She could see more clearly the differences and the similarities between the current case and her private anguish, and was freer to deal with the present clinical situation without being personally overinvolved.

* * *

As I reflect on my choice of these first two cases, I realise there is a focus on the need to give up a childlike relationship with a dead parental figure in order to understand and proceed in life. In particular, the second case represents ways of dealing with the death of an elder of the tribe. This consideration relates to the position of the Balint Society in the UK and its relationship of homage to Michael and Enid Balint as wonderful but now dead parents (Michael died in 1970 and Enid in 1996). The work that the Balints achieved for general practice in the UK and elsewhere has been immeasurable. I have no doubt, however, that, for both, the idea that the knowledge and understanding of the present generation would develop *beyond* their work would be considered the essential means for the Balint Society to stay alive and move forward, rather than remaining in a state of unconscious repetition due to an unmourned past. This is a reminder of the necessity to look ahead to the next generation, and the one beyond, bearing in mind the weight and responsibility of our history and of our learning in the overlapping area between general practice and psychoanalysis.

Case 3: addiction in the elderly

Dr C presented a case of a sweet seventy-year-old lady who was addicted to dihydrocodeine, a strong opioid analgesic. It was unclear when her addiction had begun, but it had certainly become much worse over the previous eighteen months, with the patient suffering from recurrent bouts of cold and 'flu. She was described as a tiny woman who was exceedingly thin. In addition, she complained of a terrible pain in one of her hips, yet refused to go to hospital. Eventually, the presenting doctor persuaded her and she was admitted to hospital, where the only abnormality to be found was a small amount of osteoarthritis in one of her hips. The pain that she complained about, however, was much more severe than her apparent state of health could explain.

It steadily became clear that the patient had an addictive behaviour in relation to her doctor. She would lose prescriptions, come for repeat prescriptions days earlier than when due, and would tell her doctor that she was going to visit a cousin in a distant town, and would need an extra two-weeks' supply. Dr C had recently realised, via the computer notes in the practice, that she had prescribed her patient over three thousand such analgesic tablets in the previous year, and this made her feel terrible. The patient's daughter, who was also a patient at the practice, had recently come to tell the doctor that her mother did not in fact have a cousin whom she visited. The patient had pleaded with her daughter not to tell the doctor that she had been lying, but the daughter decided that she could not possibly withhold this as she did not want to lie to her own doctor herself.

Dr C then took up a defensive position in the group, suggesting that it was perhaps best to have followed this course with the patient as she was elderly. The rest of the group were rather steely about this, commenting that the patient might have another fifteen to twenty years to live, and also wanting to consider what the patient might be like when she was not in a state of addiction. Maybe her state of mind was affecting her marriage and her relationship with her daughter, and even her grandchildren. Eventually, the doctor was able to admit that she felt very angry towards this patient for deceiving her, and that this was why she was anxious about really confronting her with her addiction. She realised that there would be a battle if she reduced the drugs by even one tablet a week. She also wondered if the patient would attend the surgery if she was challenged, as if she might become too "infirm" to travel. Addicts can move heaven and earth to get what they want. The doctor began to look rather depressed at this point.

A colleague had the idea that perhaps the doctor herself was containing and feeling the patient's depression beneath the addiction. Once it was discovered that Dr C was feeling this state of mind of her patient—causing her to be clinically stuck—she was more able to return to her usual capabilities and find her clinical direction. Dr C thought that she could take a clinical stand with this patient and slowly reduce the medication, letting both the husband and daughter, as well as her partners in the practice, know that this was going to happen, in case there was a furore. She would also try to get to know this patient better, in the expectation that, whatever her pain, its emotional significance might be discovered. Other than this clinical presentation, Dr C was not a depressed character. It was a pertinent example of a patient leaving an unconscious existence beneath the skin of the doctor, projecting aspects of their own life inside of the other. Interestingly, the group had not been told very much at all about the history or life of the patient, other than about the drugs. This was also a significant finding as, somehow, the patient had largely avoided speaking about herself, managing to make the usually competent doctor complicit in this evasion, showing no curiosity about her patient—this was despite the fact that, during her years working in the group, she consistently knew the importance of family history, and valued the stories of the early lives of her patients. This adds more weight to the idea that she was unconsciously acting as a container for aspects of her patient's mind.

Such activity may throw light on early developmental processes in the relationship between the patient, when she was a baby, and her mother. It is possible to surmise that an intense hunger for tablets to quell an addiction represented a state of emptiness in, and carried from, the early infantile life of the patient. This may further signal that Dr C was enacting the role of a distant, depressed mother. In another probable enactment, Dr C also unwittingly gave the wrong medicine to her patient, suggesting that as a baby the patient had been given things other than what was needed, such as feeding, tenderness, warmth, and authentic boundaries. Such thoughts may also connect with the initial description of her patient as being "sweet", with the possibility that she had been managed more, in her upbringing, by being given sweets, rather than something more appropriate and substantial. If so, such a hypothesis could suggest the roots of a later addiction. It would also explain the pattern of a good doctor who had unconsciously ignored her medical model with a particular patient, being unconsciously bound up in enacting an unnoticed distress. The realisation of such projections into the doctor can become the start of a real emotional engagement with the patient, even if initially, in the current case, it meant that the emotional work was embodied by a clinical fight. The work in the Balint group was not just about the doctor being told how to manage her patient, but rather gave her a sense of relief that her unconscious burden of identification with these negative aspects had been released. Through the process of noticing, feeling, and understanding these projections, Dr C was freed from the alienation that she felt from her patient.

Case 4: and a further case of addiction and neediness

The next patient, briefly discussed within the same seminar, had come to the mind of Dr D on listening to the earlier presentation. She reported the case of a woman who had had a severe breakdown in her twenties, necessitating a two-year inpatient psychiatric treatment and many weeks of sleep therapy. Since then, she had apparently been prescribed every type of psychiatric medication and, over the years, become addicted to all of them. Dr D expressed zeal about helping such a patient off their addictive medication and had done a great job, to the extent that the patient was on only one tablet at night to help her sleep, as well as a small dose of an antidepressant. The patient, beneath her presentation of addiction, seemed to have moods swinging between mania and depression. The mania she experienced was not overly extreme, and she was able to be creative with poetry and painting. In the depressive periods, however, she sought out her doctor.

Dr D described her patient as being quite childish and sensed a require-ment to mother her. Later on, when recounting the patient's history, she remembered that the patient's mother had kept her a child for too long, not wanting her to grow up. This seemed to be the doctor's transference position in relation to the patient. One member of the group wondered why the patient required any medication at all if she was in a stable state. I pointed out that the impact of continuing some tablets might be a way to keep the patient as a child to the doctor-mother and, furthermore, that it was likely that this addiction was another representation of early depriva-tion, as in Case 3. Beneath the addiction there could be a state of manic depression which, when bound or settled psychically, moved into an obses-sional state—such as the repetitive demand for drugs. If this was the patho-logical core complex, it might be necessary for the situation to be faced in the clinical encounter.

In following on from each other, these last two presentations melded in an interesting way, the latter case appearing to highlight the direction in which the first might develop. As the problem of diminishing the addiction to tablets proceeds, an addiction to a particular sort of dependent relation to the doctor is revealed. As Balint remarkably pointed out in *The Doctor, his Patient and the Illness*, the doctor *is* the medicine. The impact of the needi-ness for tablets is returned to a more primitive state of needing the doctor. How that need is manifested can then become an interesting avenue for the doctor to consider in an attempt to develop the imaginative capaci-ties of the patient. It is not so essential to spend a large amount of time with the patient here, if patients and their families can stay with the same doctor for many years. As doctors have privileged and private knowledge of internal family dynamics, they are in a powerful place to be unconsciously used when necessary.

The group meeting ended with a desire to continue looking at both of these cases of addiction at different stages of treatment, with the idea that the general practitioners had exceedingly important roles to play, involving much more than the palliation and impoverishment in the clinical relationship that the tablets imposed. The two doctors, rather than thinking formulaically, had started to become curious. There was also an understanding that such work may well be the province of ordinary medicine, instead of sending such patients to a specialist addiction service that would have hardly any knowledge of the intimate life of the patient—a life that the general practitioner, when able to transcend any projective systems, has at their fingertips.

Case 5: an emergency case

Dr E presented a case in which he found that he had been double-booked in his own practice. He was due to go to the hospital to teach on treatments for the terminally ill and, as part of the afternoon, was planning to take some time off to have a swim at the staff centre. However, he found that his receptionist had booked him to see an extra patient. He phoned the hospital and said that he would be late, which was unusual and difficult for him as he was usually assiduous in his timekeeping. He had hoped that the extra patient would not take long, but to his chagrin he then had to attend an emergency case for someone who was not even a patient of the practice.

A woman had brought her twenty-year-old nephew for an appointment. He was from the far north of the country and he immediately made it clear that he was a drug addict. The nephew had left a mental hospital despite being detained under a section of the Mental Health Act that restricted him to being an inpatient. He was demanding to be immediately prescribed Valium and other drugs. Within minutes the general practitioner found himself thoroughly angry at having to do this work, and wondered why "this chap had come all the way from the north in order to use up my time". He was internally debating whether to give him a couple of Valium tablets and send him on his way so that he could get away for his swim. At this point, the patient said, "And I've got pain in my knees, doctor." This threw the doctor, who, while thinking about what he should do, suggested that the patient should wait outside while he phoned the hospital in Scotland. The patient said, "But aren't you even going to look at my knees?" The doctor said, "What do you think the matter is?", to which the patient replied, "Well, they hurt, ever since I was crucified!" Hearing this, the doctor began to realise that the patient may well be psychotic. The patient did indeed have thoughts that he was the Son of God. The realisation came to the doctor that he was not going to get to his meeting, nor would he go swimming. The patient was starting to become quite interesting. The couple went and sat outside while the doctor rang the hospital. He discovered that the patient was a known heroin addict who had also been diagnosed as schizophrenic. He had been placed on restriction under a section of the Mental Health Act, having been notably violent in the past. The hospital was very grateful that their patient had been found, and desired that the doctor put him in the local mental hospital for twenty-four hours while they came down to collect him. The doctor then recounted this to the patient and found that he was quite pleased that he was being looked after.

What was interesting was that, despite the story of violence, the doctor had not worried about facing the patient, nor had the patient been particularly violent. It is likely that the reason was that the doctor had felt intense rage inside himself within the first three minutes of the consultation. Realising that he could do little about his lost swim he had declined to blame the patient. Otherwise, this may have lit the patient's violent fuse. Instead, in becoming interested with a patient who identified with Jesus, which was not a regular occurrence in his practice, he gave his time freely, devoting it to the clinical situation. He even had the thought of circulating to colleagues in the region that he would be very interested in dealing with psychotic drug addicts, on the condition that he had three hours free to do so!

The reason that the doctor presented this case to the group was to consider how the perception of a clinical picture is so dependent on the state of mind of the doctor. If the doctor has no space in their mind, perhaps because they are already doing something else while seeing a patient, then it is not surprising that only the surface of the situation is scratched. A diagnosis is then made, which, rather than being based on the depth of the clinical picture, fits with the doctor's preconceptions. For many, this might seem sufficient, but what is interesting is that when the doctor can deal with their own internal affective state of mind, and perhaps ambivalence—in this case, anger—then the opening up and development of the clinical picture and its good treatment—in this case, without violence—is an extraordinary outcome. Beneath the surface of a strange presentation, the patient did wish to be cared for. This is an example of a doctor being able to work with the patient by utilising their own internal state of mind, monitoring it intensely during the consultation, and overcoming their anger in order to reach a position of concern for their patient—a position that the patient might have unconsciously felt and valued.

Case 6: Whose mortality—the patient's or the doctor's?

A couple of years earlier, Mr R, now aged forty-two, had suffered a small cerebrovascular accident that had left him without the use of one arm. Otherwise, he told his doctor, he felt "as strong as a bull". He was able to function and work, and had recently painted the outside of his house. However, he had a severe cardiomyopathy, to the extent that he was only kept alive by taking medication. He had not been accepted for a heart transplant because of his earlier stroke. Dr F said that she did not know why this case had come to mind—she felt she was doing good work with the patient and his wife, even though they were both reluctant to face the serious possibility of his early death.

At her clinic she had been working on all the medical matters involved in the case, yet had suddenly discovered that the couple had attended another consultation with the new young partner in the practice. The group was told that if patients suddenly decided to change doctors within this practice the usual policy was to send them back to the original doctor. In this case, because the colleague was new, this good practice had failed to happen. Then, during the previous week, she found, again to her surprise, that the wife was now on her list wanting an urgent appointment. The wife attended by herself and spoke, with much anger, about how she wished that she would die as she felt unable to continue looking after her husband. She had recently been in anguish because, when a fifty-year-old friend had suddenly died, she had had the terrible thought of wondering why it had not been her husband instead. Some discussion went on in the group about whether the wife had unconsciously moved her husband to another doctor so that she could return to the original doctor to discuss her death wishes—and that this discussion might be very helpful. I took a different line and wondered about the lack of contact between the doctor and the new partner, but the group ignored this. Later on, I pointed out that the absence of communication between the couple, who, we had been told, did not sleep nor hug nor talk together, was now seemingly being enacted by the two doctors. Furthermore, Dr F, who was angry that the new doctor did not know the practice rules, had not spoken up to inform him. We were also told that the couple's two adult daughters sometimes made a fuss about their parents' situation, but their having left home was another source of anger for the mother as they were not present to help her look after their father. She had further imagined that they would not care for her after their father died.

At this point, the group heard that a third practice doctor had been clinically involved in a separate encounter. This further highlighted the lack of communication between the doctors in the practice. It was possible to think that the poor communication between the doctors was an enactment of a family who could only speak about their problems in a compartmentalised way. I wondered if some of the difficulty with the case was that a forty-two-year-old patient, unconsciously concerned with death, was moving to a new, younger doctor of thirty-five because of a phantasy about the vulnerability of the older doctor, who was in her sixties. Dr F had also not realised that Mrs R was concerned about her own death, but was now able to acknowledge it by remembering that, before her husband's stroke, she had suffered from a carcinoma of the breast—and, furthermore, that the lack of touch between the couple might well have stemmed from this illness, which they had never fully resolved. The doctor talked about how difficult it was looking after patients who are seriously ill or dying, yet are younger than oneself. In addition, Dr F had found that another case had come to mind of a man with a damaged arm. I felt that this thought might be connected to the fact that, at the time, I had one of my arms in a sling, due to having recently damaged my shoulder. It was becoming clear that there was a profound transference in relation to me. At the time, I was in my early forties, but perhaps in the group unconscious I was being perceived as near my death, having suffered a fracture to my body. It was important that this was exposed as an anxiety in all of us, because however much doctors may think that it is the patient who has the illness (as if we are lucky that we have got away with it), death will also come to claim us at some point. Being a doctor can sometimes provide a magical defence against fear of illness and death, as we can just project it onto our patients.

Finding such revelations about her own mortality—as well as its implications for the leader and the other members of the group—enabled Dr F to find the courage to discuss with her patients the severe illness triggering their thoughts of both death and its aftermath. This was something that she could much more easily bear to do in the knowledge that, as a result, and at some future time, she would be more able to face her own mortality. As a result of discussing this case, the doctors in the group realised that diagnosing a significant disease required them to monitor the capacities of the patient to mourn, either for the loss of bodily functioning or the approach of death itself. Practising medicine from the "cradle to the grave" means being available to help the patient bear the end of life.

It is relatively easy for the doctor to project death onto the other, yet, at times, its impact returns to unconsciously haunt the doctor, whose own mortality has to be faced. The doctor who really knows this as an important part of their own life is in a less vulnerable state with their patients who may be in the position of being unable to bear the thought of their own death. Such rejection of death can impact on the doctor, whose knowledge and proposed treatments might also be rejected by the patient. In this case, rather than feeling rejected by her patients, it was a pivotal moment of realisation for Dr F that Mr and Mrs R were unable to deal with the loss of each other. This revelation in turn helped to crystallise a deeper understanding of how the original patient, Mr R, had had to face the early loss of the object in childhood. For the analyst, areas such as the impact of early breastfeeding develop into the first loss, with the complexity of whether the breast was given up by the baby or whether the mother suddenly withdrew the object; this early loss then becomes the potential template for acceptance or disturbance around the issue of future loss. The same is true of traumatic situations, such as the premature death of a parent or sibling, and how the child managed. Whilst such matters are the natural terrain of psychoanalysis, the doctor in the Balint group may, in time, grasp some of these deep emotive structures, helping them to develop both their medical skills and the impact of such states of mind on their own character.

Case 7: waifs

Dr G reluctantly presented the case of a young woman who had left her practice some eighteen months ago. Knowing that she regarded the patient as being a very difficult character, she had also had the thought that her patient would be returning at some future time. This patient, unwanted as a child, had been brought up in a local authority home. She had married a boy who had grown up in the same home. Dr G described them as being "like a couple of waifs or strays together". She continued her description of the patient as being thin and unsavoury, and that she had two children. The patient had developed brittle diabetes, but whatever the doctor had tried—being kind, being firm, pointing out the dangerousness of the patient's carelessness, every modality she could think of—her patient declined to take her diabetic medication. In addition, the doctor had taken a vaginal smear that was found to be abnormal, and the patient needed to return to the clinic for further investigation. The patient could not be found, however—she had just disappeared. The doctor had been very concerned about the dangerous implications of the result of the smear—not only for the patient, but also for her children. With much concern, Dr G told the group that nothing she had done with this particular patient had ever helped. The patient had disappeared, her husband was in trouble with the police, and Dr G thought that these events had something to do with the breakup of the marriage. However, a letter had then been received at the practice from the young woman, asking if she could return as a patient. The group wondered if the patient was applying to have Dr G as her doctor again, or somebody else in the practice. Unhesitatingly, Dr G thought it was an invitation to return to her. The group generally took quite a tough attitude towards this patient, and various doctors thought that she should first be invited to return for an initial interview to see if she was now going to be a compliant patient. Gradually, however, Dr G began to warm up from her initial antipathy and slowly began to realise that she quite liked this woman, despite her difficult character. She found she was even looking forward to seeing her old patient, and was very surprised at discovering this change in her own attitude.

One way of thinking about the story was that the couple, without parents, had been like babes in the woods. The doctor could function as a wicked witch, offering the woman nice sweets to help her diabetes, but the patient regarded the medication offered as poisonous and wanted nothing to do with it. The significance of re-finding the doctor again was that it enabled the patient to have an experience, perhaps for the first time in her life, of returning and finding a parent who had not disappeared but was still present. This was seen as a creative opportunity, as long as the doctor could allow it to develop and not be prejudiced by the manner of the patient's earlier sudden departure. It was the negative imagination of the presenting doctor that affected her opinion of the case, which concluded with Dr G being delighted to find that there was a basis for creatively renewing her care for this particular patient. For the doctor, the possibility of still being present and available for the patient, who had grown up with no expectation that someone would be there for her, was a potentially remarkable new state. The case was one that was predicated on loss, with the patient unconsciously expecting, from long experience, that she—and her "sibling" husband—were alone. Yet there remained enough hope in the patient to expect the object to still be there on her return. The patient's psychic system demanded to be tested, and luckily, whilst the doctor felt the emotional impact of the departure of her patient, she was able to not retaliate. This allowed the object to survive and be found by the returning patient.

The character of the doctor

To only consider the effect on the clinical encounter of the particularities of the patient is not quite accurate enough, however, as different doctors respond very differently to the same clinical situation. We must return to the territory of the character and personality of the individual doctor, and their impact on her or his medicine. Whilst working in a Balint group does not demand that participants have an analysis, it is an expectation that some parts of their characters, in the context of the clinical work, will need to be explored within the privacy of the group. Balint expected that participants would go through a character development in order that they would be more aware of their psychic responsibilities within the clinical encounter. The doctor stuck with the heart-sink patient will often need to find new emotional resources within themselves in order to become available in a new way with their patient. This is very different from the doctor being given a prescription from the group, in a way that a patient often expects to receive a prescription from their doctor in place of something more tangibly complex.

Case 8: homosexual anxiety in the doctor

A doctor presented a case in the Balint group concerning his perplexity over a recent clinical encounter. He had been attending a home visit to a patient and just as he was arriving he saw the local priest, who he knew and who was also his patient. They stopped for a brief chat. The priest was about to go on a foreign holiday and spoke about his impending trip with much enthusiasm. He said he was going to attend the surgery as he wanted a 'flu jab in order to protect himself from illness. As he lived a few doors along the street and the doctor had the injection in his bag, Dr J suggested that he could call round in a little while as he was so close by, and this offer was accepted enthusiastically. Fifteen minutes later, Dr J went over to the priest's house and, to his surprise, found that the front door was ajar. It was the first time he had made a home visit there. He called out to his patient that he had arrived, and was a little surprised when the patient shouted out for the doctor to enter his house and come upstairs, where he was waiting in the bedroom. The doctor felt somewhat confused as he had expected to go into the living room, and with his patient's sleeve rolled up give a subcutaneous injection into the upper arm. In a matter of two or three minutes he could then have given the treatment and returned to his office. His sense of uncertainty grew as he climbed the stairs. The bedroom door was ajar and he could see the pink hue of the wallpaper. On entering he found the patient fully naked, face down on the pink-sheeted bed, saying, "Doctor, give it to me in my bottom." Dr J felt extremely uncomfortable, said the injection was for the patient's arm, gave it very quickly, and found himself fleeing from the house. Once back in his office his disturbance continued, but in a somewhat unprocessed way. He felt very uncertain about what had happened but he knew that he was very upset about the encounter.

The other doctors in the group were smiling by now, and there was a general sense of amusement in the room, which further perplexed Dr J. The other doctors in the group were aware that the priest was making a seductive play for the doctor, and were clear that the patient was homosexual and had planned that the "medical" encounter would take place in the seductive intimacy of his pink bedroom—naked, exposing his bottom, and asking for penetration through the cipher of an injection. This was all readily understood by the other doctors in the group. Dr J began to move from a feeling of perplexity to a mixture of being annoyed and embarrassed in the group. In fact, the clinical difficulty seemed to be less the patient's behaviour and more the doctor's response. It was as if he was humiliated by the thought that he too was homosexual, and that all of the doctors in the group knew it, other than him. He was mollified when I pointed out that the story could be seen to describe a doctor being homosexually assaulted out of the blue. But now he felt very angry, especially as his offer to save his patient the time of attending and waiting at the practice was treated with such disregard and disdain. He thought of barring the patient from the practice, as he felt that he never wanted to see him again. Gradually, though, he realised that retaliation would be too much of a counterattack, devoid of understanding. The group decided that in future it would be clinically appropriate for all consultations with that patient to take place within the formal confines of the doctor's office. Often, the context of the clinical encounter requires firm boundaries. In this case the patient would be likely to be better able to contain his sexual excitement in the doctor's surgery than in his own seductively pink bedroom.

This example examines the difficulty of a doctor's character in a particular clinical moment. Dr J was unaware of the homosexuality of his patient. Other doctors may also not know about some aspects of their patients' sexual lives, but the doctors in the Balint group—albeit from an easier position of hearing the encounter at a distance—had a clear understanding of the patient's seduction of his doctor. Dr J was unaware of this, and perhaps this was a result of his own uncertainty about himself. This is a topic that is of less interest to Balint groups, which do not function in order to offer psychoanalysis to their members. However, in this case, the doctor's own sexuality was a crucial element in understanding his perplexity. The important fact was not that his patient became a different character from the chaste priest he had imagined, but rather that the doctor's own psychosexual position did not allow him the flexibility of thought to perceive what all the other doctors immediately understood. Dr J left the group with more understanding of his patient, but also with a glimmer of knowledge about a private area of himself—implicitly revealed to him through the new experience of discussing his difficulty in recognising his patient's homosexual enactment. This case demonstrates both the diverse uses that can be made of the doctor and the value of the doctor having the freedom to understand more of their own private prejudices, rather than allowing them to hinder their clinical freedom.

At another level of understanding, however, the encounter revealed a priest who may have been moving towards being sexually out of control. The seductive enactment with the doctor could then be something to work with at a later time, in order to establish whether the patient was aware of his violation of ordinary professional boundaries with his excited sexual behaviour. At a time when so many priests fail in this area of life, the clinical vignette has a poignancy concerning whether an eruption of sexual desire at the wrong time, and with the wrong person, could later be examined in a consultation, the doctor investigating his concerns about the psychosexual problems of his patient in his priestly life—indicated by his overt enactment of coercive and promiscuous behaviour. For this, the doctor would need a certain bravery, based on his own sense of himself, including his sexual self. The doctor has to first identify with his patient as being in a state of provocative seduction, and then to return to his own self in order to be able to process what has happened. This is the same mental trajectory of identifications as for the psychoanalyst. The next consultation discussing the behaviour might be one that could prevent a severe acting out by the priest in his community, with the possibility of both harming himself and distressing others.

The analyst neither conducts home visits nor touches their patients, other than shaking hands occasionally, which can then assume an important evocation. In the handshake, the patient places themselves in the analyst's hands. In a way, the doctor's privileged position of sometimes going to the home—witnessing the atmosphere, colours, smells, pictures and effects—with its visual and sensual representation, allows a deep unconscious awareness of the other. Very often, being in the room of their patient is greatly evocative, and has an equivalence with the patient being in the mind of the analyst. This is even truer of the doctor's privileged position in relation to the body of their patient. In the current case, instead of the priest bringing concerns about his sexual life to the doctor they were enacted between them in the intimacy of the patient's home. The doctor was not there to enact back to the patient, but rather this was perhaps the only way that the patient could bring his own distress about his sense of a perhaps disinhibited desire. From this perspective, Dr J's perplexity could be understood as a projection onto him of his patient's non-understanding of the potential impact of his sexuality on the rest of his life—an important subject in the life of his patient and a far more complex position than just a rather odd form of seduction. Of course, it was up to Dr J, having learnt from his case that his initial incomprehension signalled the emergence of an anxiety around his own unconscious homosexuality, whether this would be an issue he might want to understand more about in the privacy of his own therapy.

There are great possibilities for reciprocal learning in the Balint group. The doctor can, of course, learn how psychoanalysts think and talk about the clinical encounter. We scrutinise every detail of the patient's communications, verbal and non-verbal; what is spoken, and what is not. Psychoanalysts can also learn from doctors about how they can be used as a substrate on which patients etch their unconscious object relationships. Both patients' homes and bodies can be active in the enactments of these relationships, in a way that the analyst, because of the structure and boundaries of the analytic method, must discover in more roundabout ways, through the imagination and free association. For both doctor and analyst there is great value in listening to the complex rhythms of the psyche-soma, and in giving equal and serious attention to minute details in the doctor–patient relationship.

Doctors and psychoanalysts: Medical freedom and Balint's tradition

We get tiny little important details which really make the thing alive for the patient, and then, once you do that, the patient tells you something different and unexpected. That is the transference in the true sense, not just in the "here and now".

(Enid Balint, 1993, p. 223)

Perseus wore a magic cap that the monsters he hunted down might not see him. We draw the magic cap down over eyes and ears as a make-believe that there are no monsters.

(Karl Marx, 1867, p. xviii)

The ethos of *The Doctor, his Patient and the Illness* is presently undergoing a substantial attack within the so-called rationalistic evidence-based medicine that is sweeping through clinical practice in both the UK and other countries. On the surface, the doctor's attention appears to be directed towards more modern medical practices, enlisting evincing evidence that has been carefully measured, evaluated, and controlled in trials. The assumption is that this is something new and that doctors have only recently been thoughtful about the scientific basis of medical practice. Yet it is hard to find evidence for this as, to my knowledge, doctors have always examined the clinical evidence prior to making a therapeutic decision. Evidence-based medicine has positive associative links to state-of-the-art scientific experiments, high-technology medical evaluation, and large double-blind trials. The present-day medical empiricism, taking evidence from an existing order of things—which, as such, are often easily measured—is inherently prone to accepting as realities things that are merely evidence of underlying biases and ideological pressures. Such medicine also has a negative association, however, in that it often appears to discard the evidence of the doctor's own clinical evaluation—in the old-fashioned sense of examining the patient, looking with care, and seeing the signs and symptoms that the non-doctor fails to notice. Valuable clinical evidence can be derived from the examination of one's own practice over many years.

The insidious underbelly of this new trend is less about clinical confidence and "correct" diagnosis than the saving of money. It emanates from the world of business, generated by the medical insurance complex—who want to control the industry of medicine for profit—and helped along by a willing government, keen to reduce the cost of healthcare. If medicine can be commercialised in a more orderly way, such as the dispatch of the same items of clinical treatment again and again (like the simple production and consumption of baked beans or fizzy drinks), then its cost base can be more easily rationalised and more clearly defined. Such business control creates the expectation of profits or savings to follow. In order for this to happen, doctors (who are not businessmen) need to be controlled so that they follow particular known patterns—a sort of medical factory mentality. If all doctors and patients can be forged together in a finite number of evidences, then the whole system can be "efficiently" and profitably run. All one needs to do is to leave out the individuality of the doctor and the patient, and the relationship of this individuality to a particular illness. Of course, there is plenty of evidence for the importance of considering these aspects of treatment in its evaluation. But for "insurance-based medicine"—as I will now refer to evidence-based medicine—this is a lesser part of the picture. Certainly, the character of the doctor and the patient, within their clinical relationship, can only impede the easy running of such a business. The therapeutic ideas established by Balint in his groups have to be ignored precisely because they expose insurance-based medicine as having too simplistic a logic. This may lead, for instance, to the mentally ill needing to have so-called "rationalised" care. Many insurance companies now decide that six sessions of psychological therapy is the treatment limit for most mental illness, and this is to be provided by psychiatrists and psychologists rather than qualified psychotherapists, let alone psychoanalysts. What can be special about the number six, other than its small size? Under the guise of evidence, which actually does not exist, commercialisation is turning its back on appropriate, well-tried treatment—which then becomes further ignored by young doctors because of this rejection by the present healthcare industry. However, even a year's psychodynamic psychotherapy may save many more years of costly inpatient treatment in the future. A recovered young person may, after such real therapy, attend university, obtain a job, and, in time, be able to pay taxes. These elements are not part of the calculations, nor is the quotient of internal happiness and its further impact on future family life. A business model does not include this kind of medical equation as it is dominated by the current year's expenditure and how this can be reduced. In addition, many people are more comfortable with counsellors and therapists who are not analytically trained, and are often suspicious of psychoanalysts—like the patient's wife in the second vignette, they perhaps feel that psychoanalysts may bring mess into the house.

How does one begin to understand the simplistic meaning of empiricist medical evidence when it involves the complexity of human beings, rather than machines? In such a system, the relationship between the doctor and the patient is ignored as if irrelevant. The power of the pill or medical procedure, rather than the value of the clinical relationship, appears to be the only factor behind success (or failure). Within the current trend, altering diagnoses and sudden changes of medication become the totality of the medical picture. By examining the relationship between doctor and patient, the above vignettes evidence that there is much to be noted in the undersurface of the clinical story. Putting this relationship at the centre of clinical medicine offers a deeper and more thoughtful professional activity than just relying on textbook method.

Let us revisit the first two cases from the previous chapter. What happened in them? The first, in particular, is one that had cost the NHS a great deal of money due to the way that evidence seemed to have been misunderstood. As we saw, the doctor was haunted by observations from her student days that had continued to exist within her as unresolved mourning. In the second case, the doctor was able to make a conscious connection between a painful area of privacy, of the self and her private relationships, and its clash with and reactivation in the context of the present clinical case. As often occurs in life, we suffer from the return, in the present time, of some painful past experience. If it has never been properly psychically digested it can remain, awaiting an attachment to the present world, in order, perhaps, that the ghost can at last be laid to rest. The doctor is not obtaining a surreptitious analysis within the Balint group, but there can be no deep understanding of the clinical situation without an unconscious understanding of their character within the clinical relationship under observation. The first case developed the theme of something left behind from medical training. An earlier experience, which related to whether the doctor can be a hero or can be destructive, had emerged in a new form. This obstructed the ordinary, procedural need of speaking doctor-to-doctor about a case, and interfered with the atmosphere necessary for a candid medical decision about treatment. For this, the doctor had to re-establish that she had the necessary adult skills herself, rather than being the student observer of the life and death struggle, which was not an appropriate position for her clinical work. In the second case, meanwhile, there was a confluence of connections between a family dealing with a dying father and husband and its private meaning for the doctor, which was standing in the way of her usual good medical practice. Yet the depth of both of these cases is very difficult to understand unless we accept unconscious processes and the free-association methodology derived from psychoanalytic theory and treatment. It is difficult to conceive of such complex, unconscious states of mind, deeply embedded within the core identity and character structure of each individual doctor, as being part of the new wave of evidence-based medicine. The second clinical case was suffused with unconscious processes within the doctor. This observation is not merely an interesting insight; it is an observation that enabled the individual doctor to more carefully and successfully treat her patient. Within the safety and holding of the Balint group it does not take a long time to explore such private and inner matters and, once explained, it is not difficult to understand the complexity of mixing present and past. Yet resistance to knowledge of the internal, unconscious processes of a doctor is often great, and instead we are offered the one-dimensional mode of "external", physical evidence. Knowledge of that external evidence, when combined with a developed awareness of the internal state of mind causing the doctor's stuckness in treating their patient, becomes a more powerful tool.

The Balint group can be that rare place in which this important piece of care—for the doctor and of the doctor—can be processed. Slowly, carefully, a process of unconscious interaction can be seen. Occasionally, one can see a turning point in the doctor's medical developmental history, particularly around a point of arrested affect. And, indeed, as this clinical work is based on the ordinary scientific platform of observation, discussed within the group, and linking the past clinical work with the present clinical difficulties, who can say that this is not truly evidence-based medicine?

* * *

With the apparent knowledge that its methodology is sound, medicine can retreat to an inner citadel—we can possess an inner freedom of spirit, even while we suffer from mere external tyranny. But today, like psychoanalysis, and for similar reasons, general medical practice is under threat. As Isaiah Berlin put it in his "Two concepts of liberty" (1958, p. 229), a negative liberty is expanded when nobody stops us from doing what we want, and is reduced when somebody does. I can see plenty of merit for describing the present direction of governmental meddling with medical politics as being authoritarian and against the freedom of the doctor to practise their own competent medicine. In opposition to this trend, the Balint group approach to clinical medicine has a precious possession—a medical freedom, based on free association in respect of a process called unconscious thought, derived from psychoanalytic theory. This is the value of the input from psychoanalysis in relation to general practice, and it seems clear that if the link with psychoanalysis becomes further attenuated the clarity of its usefulness may well diminish.

Like psychoanalysis, the concept of whole-body medicine, including the mind as the link between psyche and soma, humanises medicine. Such a humanising function is particularly needed in our world of specialties, part-body functions, technologies, and technocrats, all of which have an overall effect of reducing our humanness and humanity to a particular, correct status. I do not intend to contrast one approach as "good" and the other as "bad". Medical freedom needs to encompass the valued practice of both clinical positions—Balint's whole-person-centred medicine and the super-specialties of particular scientific evidences. It is the entwining of the two approaches that makes for the best of medical practice: science with humanity, practised with freedom. Thus, the wisest course is for the doctor to feel free to practise the medicine that is theirs to practise. This may seem an obvious statement, yet in these times when the trend points towards the formulaic, specific items of clinical service (the near-exact evidential occurrence), the doctor's freedom to practise is their only defence against becoming an automatic technologist. What technologist would not pause for a moment at the interesting stories that we are privileged to hear and speak of in our medical practices, and would not be thoughtful about what we do?

CHAPTER FOUR

The psychoanalyst and the psychiatric clinic

At any street corner the feeling of absurdity can strike any man in the face.

—Albert Camus, *The Myth of Sisyphus* (1942, p. 16)

Freud's prediction that the "large-scale application" of psycho-analysis must force us to "alloy the pure gold of analysis freely with the copper of direct suggestion" was followed by the comment that "whatever form this psychotherapy for the people may take, whatever the elements out of which it is compounded, its most effective and most important ingredients will assuredly remain those borrowed from strict and untendentious psycho-analysis" (Freud, 1919a, p. 168). But how is the psychoanalyst to behave in the confused world beyond the comfort of their analytic consulting room?

The psychoanalyst, as consultant psychotherapist in a psychiatric clinic or hospital setting, is invited to train staff as psychotherapists, as well as to help them in the acquisition of psychodynamic skills in order that they are more psychologically competent in their particular fields. The same may be true for social workers, occupational therapists, nurses, general practitioners, and psychologists—those members of the helping professions that work with the psychotherapist in the mental hospital. The role for the consultant is specifically focused on helping these professionals be better at their own jobs—with all the clinical, interpersonal human relationships involved—rather than on training them as specialist psychotherapists or psychoanalysts. The problem that presents itself is how to train staff who deal with patients' psychological problems to be aware of and sensitive to unconscious processes without offering them the well-proven method of going through personal analysis themselves. This difficulty is compounded by the fact that, whilst training is not a substitute for the staff's own therapy, there is often a pull towards covertly obtaining such personal therapy.

A person's awareness of the unconscious is altered little by lectures, seminars, or even the supervision of case material, other than in an intellectual and usually highly defended modality. Unless, of course, this is accompanied by their own psychotherapeutic experience. Otherwise, what is usually missing is an inner experience of a conviction in the role of the unconscious in the dynamic process. The pressure to teach in this intellectual and academic way is usually significant. An institution such as a psychiatric department expects lectures, and the trainees expect supervision and seminars. All of this can be unconsciously designed to neutralise the psychoanalyst in the institutional setting. Arguably, as long as the psychoanalyst is mainly addressing these institutional pressures and "needs", they are directed into only being a psychotherapist for the staff—and as a consequence become merely a castrated psychoanalyst. For the psychiatric establishment, it may be proper for the psychotherapist to provide knowledge on various topics. And as long as it stays in the form of lectures and seminars it may be safe, neutralised, and reasonably harmless—certainly away from the vicissitudes and depth of the clinical relationship.

The various techniques of psychotherapy offer the developing therapist a variety of defensive possibilities—partial solutions to their own unconscious conflicts, or an efficient repository of narcissistic supplies. However, whilst the trainee may certainly gain a great deal from being an active and magically omnipotent therapist, the possibility of that student working through their conflicts within their own treatment is usually slim. Should the trainee be satisfied with the use they make of various psychotherapeutic techniques, which may help both patients and themselves but which are often external, tacked-on skills—sometimes a type of character armour? Or is there a possibility that the psychoanalyst might be able to effect an internal change in the student—one which is then the driving force for their development of psychodynamic skill?

It is very difficult to maintain an analytic stance in such psychiatric clinics as one is likely to be seen by non-analytic colleagues (psychotherapists and psychiatrists) as being awkward, perhaps not fitting in with departmental life. This awkwardness is not something to be avoided, however. In the same way that a patient would not be encouraged to neutralise analytic work, why should the same responsibility be evaded in a position as a consultant in an institution? Whilst it is not the fault of colleagues that they too have an unconscious which gives them capacity for resistance, it is this factor that needs to be kept constantly under consideration, in order that the psychoanalyst can develop an analytic relation to the psychiatric institution. This can often become a battle over the need for this psychoanalytic way of thinking, obstacles being thrown at the psychoanalyst such as the expectation that they be on call for hospital emergencies throughout the day, thus disrupting their clinical sessions, or the expectation that they present theories of psychodynamics and the complexities of the mind in the same brief way that behavioural techniques are taught. Another attack on thinking would be an invitation to supervise psychotherapy trainees once monthly on patients seen once every two weeks. In response to these strategies, the analyst must construct their boundaries with care, opposing onslaughts on their professional life yet also trying to take their colleagues along with their strange analytic behaviour. The alternative is to submit to their pressure, and there resides, I would argue, the demise of the analyst in the hospital setting.

One way to give a psychiatric resident trainee real inside experience of the analytic relationship is to establish an analytic stance with them oneself, yet keeping to a boundary of not being their analyst. The consultant psychoanalyst can create an analytic setting in which the trainee can observe to a certain extent how analysts behave and talk, and, more importantly, can become acquainted with their ways of thinking. An important part of this is the maintenance of a quiet atmosphere, in which the psychoanalyst can listen with a free-floating mind, tolerating and even sometimes welcoming silences. Time is given to find out what is being thought, and for ideas to develop and expand, with boundaries of starting and ending the supervision without being interrupted being essential—such work should certainly not be undertaken in discussions in corridors in between other tasks.

Some of the following theoretical ideas about training mental health professionals are derived from Enid and Michael Balint's general practitioner seminars, as well as from the Hungarian system of analysis. The British system of analytic training followed that described in Berlin with the tripartite model—that is, personal analysis, theoretical courses, and protracted analytic clinical work under supervision, all kept separately from one another. In the Berlin system, when the countertransference of the candidate to their patient comes up in work under supervision, it is, by tacit agreement, not dealt with in that environment but is instead left to be worked through in the personal analysis. Thus, the emphasis in supervision is focused on the understanding of the particulars of the patient's psychodynamics, and is usually taken from the stance of "what does the patient try to convey to their analyst?" The Hungarian analytic training added the extra possibility that the candidate's personal analyst carries out one of the supervisions of the candidate's cases. To quote Michael Balint:

> In the Hungarian system, the interrelation of the transference of the patient and the counter-transference of his analyst is in the focus of attention right from the start, and remains there. What is studied is the interaction of these two transferences, that is, how they influence and modify each other.
>
> (M. Balint, 1957, p. 299)

This is the experience that Balint used to develop a training based chiefly on the close study, by group methods, of the worker's countertransference—that is, Balint groups. Sheilagh Davies and I began the first Balint group for psychiatrists in training at the Royal Free Hospital in 1980. Soon after, I established such groups outside London, following my own appointment as consultant psychotherapist. As I have described, the aim for Balint in his general practitioner groups was to develop in the doctors a sensitivity to the patient's emotional problems, thus enabling them to understand these problems more safely and in greater depth, and to use this understanding for therapeutic effect. Again, it is important to note that *"the acquisition of psychotherapeutic skills does not consist only of learning something new: it inevitably also entails a limited, though considerable, change in the doctor's personality"* (M. Balint, 1957, p. 299, italics in original). The effectiveness of using Balint groups with psychiatrists depends on their capacity to notice and tolerate emotional factors active in their patients that they rejected or ignored before, and to learn to accept these as worthy of attention.

The internal states of mind of patients in the mental hospital, together with their impact on the staff, are clinical matters that are far too often ignored or considered as irrelevant. Such resistance is projected into the readily accepted "medical model" of seeing illness as biochemical, behavioural, and in need of drug treatment such that discourse about history and feelings is regarded as minor or irrelevant. In addition, junior psychiatrists treat more severely ill patients—usually, but not only, those diagnosed with depression—and have to give electroconvulsive treatment (ECT), prescribed by their consultant, together with an anaesthetist. Whilst this treatment has been in use since the 1930s there is no real theoretical explanation offered to its application. Yet it is a treatment that finds the psychiatrist applying a severe electric shock such that it is hard for the doctor not to be perceived, or to perceive themselves, as being aggressive towards the patient—especially with electrocution's links to torture. It is unsurprising that some patients try to avoid staff out of fear.

There are important differences to note in the use of Balint groups in mental hospitals—with the staff working in them—compared with general practice. In the Balint group, psychiatric trainees can be given an attenuated form of psychoanalysis that can make them think, "Yes, why didn't I think of this?" or, "Why did I rush on by and leave such and such out?" or, "Why did I not have the courage to take my strange thoughts about the clinical interaction more seriously?" The use of countertransference and analytic understanding can reveal a paradox or lacuna, a presence or an absence in the clinical relationship. This in itself can be realised as being highly unusual by those trainees whose expectation of a medical system is that it is solely interested in labels and formulaic diagnoses, and in responding with the prescription of psychotropic drugs. There is often something in the doctor themselves deriving support from this usual psychiatric way of working. If this can be glimpsed by the doctor then their embrace of the organic and the known may be disrupted, allowing them to direct their attention—in the course of work with patients, but also, in so doing, with themselves—to the fearful, the unknown, the paradoxical, and the fragmented. There is also then a chance that, following such experiences, some participants realise the effectiveness of psychoanalysis and wish to further develop themselves by undergoing a personal analysis.

Only occasionally can the psychoanalyst have such an impact on a doctor, however. One is usually working with doctors and nurses with high levels of scepticism and resistance, and sometimes psychiatrically ill colleagues. Sometimes, perhaps, the awfulness of what a colleague is doing to a patient—for example, when a doctor is projecting their illness onto an ill patient—is too much to bear, even for the insightful colleague. This is a subject that patients are often well aware of, such that they do not say more about their symptoms if they think that the doctor cannot bear to hear it. It is well known that in the profession of psychiatry there is a high level of mentally ill or characterologically disturbed individuals who prefer to maintain the illusion that the illness is to be found in the patient, rather than in themselves; that is, their being a psychiatrist is operating as a convenient way of hiding from their self. In these cases, the Balint group can sometimes be supportive to the ill doctor, and at the same time relieve the patient of the burden. The psychoanalyst leading the group may be able to ease the doctor towards having their own personal analysis in some separate place. If not, though, one has to suffer the frustration of being impotent in such circumstances, remaining the voyeur of poor practice. This is a painful problem for the trainer. There may be many indications that a colleague is practising a rigid, defensive psychiatry, projecting pathological parts of themselves onto the patient. Ideally, as already suggested, the analyst may act to hold more of the pathological projections, relieving the patient of such burdens. Other psychiatrists in the group can also be helpful and supportive to an ill colleague.

Like the method of Balint groups with general practitioners, those with junior psychiatrists do not focus on the psychotherapy cases themselves, in isolation, but rather on the everyday work that the psychiatrist does with their patient—the task is not general supervision but rather to focus on the problem that the doctor has with their patient. This aim of this method is to enable the participants to feel the emotional impact of their everyday clinical relationships, as well as to make sense of the interactive processes in terms of psychoanalytic theory. The participant's experience of their everyday work as trainees can often be more dominated by "learning to do what the supervisor does", however. In these cases, one can see the development of formulaic, rote skills through mimesis rather than through a real inner learning experience, alive with conviction. After some time, though, many doctors attending the seminar begin to obtain a feeling for the material of their patient's cases in terms of the latter's past life and experiences. I do not mean this in a flat, unemotional, correct, psychiatric history, but through experiencing the past relationships of the patient within the presenting illness, as well as in the "here and now" transference of the patient–doctor relationship. Here there can be a living transferential relationship, and the doctor, once they have begun to experience such feelings in themselves, about their work with the patient, has been able to shift inside of themselves how they function as a psychiatrist.

Clinical vignettes of Balint groups with psychiatrists

Case 1: the anorexic group

After several months, two of the doctors attending the Balint group became responsible for the inpatient group of anorexic patients in the hospital. One session of that group of patients was described in which all of them complained about how precisely the correct amount of potato should be placed on the plate at mealtimes. The discussion in the Balint group then developed into how precise the words used by the hospital staff, as a whole, had to be. "The staff should use neither too many nor too few words in communicating with the anorexic patients, but just sufficient." All of the staff should be given lists of words that should or should not be said, as they had been saying upsetting things such as "Now you are looking better." The group then began to discuss the links which can be seen between behaviour, verbal language, and thinking, and to notice the same mental mechanisms present in the group of anorexics, preoccupied on the surface with their bodies and their weight. The seminar became silent for a moment, and then quite excited, it gradually being realised that external behaviour was an expression of internal thought and fantasy that the doctors could then think about. This was far different from the commencement of the case discussion, in which it was felt that the patients' thoughts and talk was irrelevant—the doctors having been taught that anorexia was a problem of brain pathology, making listening superfluous. In the ensuing discussion the doctors began to recognise a pattern between the pathology of anorexia and the pattern of eating, and furthermore to then find the same pattern in their relationships with the hospital staff, and in the transference—the doctors' anxiety over precision in communicating with patients mimicking the latter's concern over the specifications of their food. Moreover, the type of dialogue unconsciously expected by the patients seemed to be one in which one person would be ruthlessly in control. And so, with the patients taking such a position over the specifications of their food, the doctors realised that their own sense of helplessness before these strictures may reflect an earlier sense of great vulnerability in the face of an extremely critical, demanding, or controlling parent. This underlying commentary could be given attention rather than regarded as chatter, understood, and used by the doctors in their treatment by relating to their patients in a new way—by realising the value of listening.

Case 2: one of us is cut off

A young woman who had taken a severe overdose, and survived, had told everyone around her that everything was now all right. Soon after, she took another overdose and was brought into hospital against her wishes, under a section of the Mental Health Act. She continued to persuade anyone in the hospital who would listen to her that she was actually well. After being precipitously discharged she again overdosed, and was again brought back to the same hospital. Sometime later, the patient was once more discharged, and the junior doctor seeing her in the outpatient department presented on her in the seminar. Dr K did not know what he could do. He referred her for a psychotherapy consultation but she did not attend. "She is so cut off", he said. One member of the group remembered that the previous time the doctor had presented this patient was when she had been an inpatient. He had brought the problem of what to do with an importuning patient, describing how she continually tugged on his sleeve when she found him in the corridor, asking if she could leave as she was now fine. He had also related how she would wear a provocative nightgown, expressly denying being depressed or ill. What he had been describing seemed to have been felt by him as an attack by his patient to the extent that it severely curtailed his movements on the ward, in fear of being met and overwhelmed by her demands. What was extraordinary, however, was Dr K's total denial of this memory, even though it was clearly remembered by the other seminar members. He wanted to move on quickly and was irritated with us that we were wasting time with irrelevant things. In doing so, it seemed apparent that he wanted to deny the patient her madness, along with the impact of this madness on himself.

Rather than quickly passing on to other matters, Dr K was instead invited to look at his apparent memory loss. After a few moments' pause he rediscovered the memory. He said it was true: he had forgotten how provocative she had been towards him. On thinking more, he was able to realise the strangeness of his memory lapse, as at the time she had had a very powerful effect on him. I then said: "The patient does not acknowledge a state of mind such as depression and suicidalness, and is cut off from it. Perhaps you are in identification with your patient so that you cannot remember the ill part of her attacking you (or revealing itself to you). This would be in order to make it apparently easier for you to see your patient in the outpatient department and say, 'It's all OK.'" The group was particularly struck by this, and there was a realisation of the degree to which the powerful patient was influencing the doctor's thinking. This enabled Dr K to grasp the material more completely, and, with renewed freedom to think, he was able to work in a new way with his patient, rather than being mimetic.

This doctor had a capacity to think and to feel. He talked carefully and thoughtfully about the omnipotence of doctors, the medical hierarchy, and organic psychiatry. He also related how he had thought about embarking on psychotherapy training, yet confessed to the group that now he felt quite lost and unsure about the idea. In this state of being lost, however, he had still had the capacity to present his work honestly, and to accept the group's thoughts. The group was a point in his development where the thinking and the feeling of his general psychiatric work could become connected.

Case 3: suicide

Dr L had missed the session the week before as she had had to deal with the aftermath of the suicide of one of her inpatients. At the next meeting she began to talk about the young male patient, who had killed himself by jumping in front of a train. She wondered anxiously what could have been done to stop the suicide, and decided that the patient should have had ECT. Apparently, other patients on the ward had known of his intentions, and he had tried to kill himself some time earlier, when on a walk away from the ward. It was the other patients that had managed to dissuade him from harming himself at that time. Dr L also thought that the patient had not been on special observation—that is, allocated an individual nurse—as there was an acute shortage of nurses on the ward. The nurses on the ward, when they heard the news of the death of a patient, had suggested to the doctor that there ought to be a community ward meeting to break the news to the other patients. Dr L was most reluctant and only agreed with much trepidation. She acknowledged her fantasy that, if told, the other patients would follow suit and kill themselves.

In terms of her knowledge of her patient, the doctor could give only a fragmentary history. He had been admitted following problems with his job. He was an agricultural graduate who had apparently felt unwanted in his present employment. His mother had recently married for a second time, to an electrician. In addition to this, his intended move away from home had collapsed. The patient subsequently became very lively, noisy, and disruptive at home, against his usually very quiet nature. His mother's concern led to his admission to the hospital, where the psychiatrist had diagnosed the patient as having a "situational crisis". On questioning for more details by the group it emerged that, following his mother's new marriage, he had been invited to leave the house—his home. The group then learnt that the patient's father had killed himself when the patient was fifteen years old, wrapping wire around his body and electrocuting himself. This fact was provided in a desultory way, as though it was hardly worth mentioning. The group then heard that at admission the young man had been given a diagnosis of mania—which was "obvious", according to his doctor. "What else could be done?" she said. Clearly there was much confusion over the diagnosis. There followed a silence. I asked about the community meeting, as it had been mentioned but not discussed; she said it had gone well enough. The patients had supported the staff and told them that they were not to blame. Of course, we were told, that only happened after the psychotic female patient had been removed. The group smiled but was not curious. It was as if the utterances of patients, especially mad patients, were irrelevant to understanding and need not be listened to. I asked why someone had to be removed in order for the meeting to work. I was wondering what the thing was that had to be repudiated—banished from the room. We were told that the psychotic patient had told the meeting that she was the angel of death and that others in the room would follow this death (interestingly, this seemed to be the same unacceptable thought that the doctor herself had had, and which demanded being shut out of her own mind). She also said that she would have wished to push the patient in front of the train herself. Nurses then removed the patient, apparently in order to allow the community meeting to be supportive to the staff. Nobody in the Balint group wanted to make anything of these interesting statements and the conversation turned back to organic methods of treatment and the value of ECT in endogenous depression. After a while I said that it could be helpful to think that the idea of suicide might be seen to contain its opposite, the unconscious wish to murder, turned against the self to perhaps protect the object of the murderous desire from hatred. This is an example of the unconscious operation of an opposite as a disguise for a wish, similar in concept to a mania which has, as its hidden opposite, a depressive state. It seemed that the reason that the psychotic patient who had suggested murder—with the phantasy of herself pushing the patient in front of a train—had to be excluded from everyone else was because her murderous suggestion echoed a similar wish on the part of the patient. Essentially, this argument rests on the idea that a suicidal attack on the self, however awful, is easier to accept than the hatred bound up in the wish to kill the other.

Dr L then remembered that the patient had killed himself on his mother's birthday. A great sigh of knowingness then went around the group. Now sense could begin to be made of the fragmented history. It could be imagined that the patient's suicide was a birthday present for his mother, an expression of rage and hatred that he felt for her. Her remarrying had certainly led to the marked possibility of his exclusion from his home, which is likely to have profoundly upset the patient. His suicide could now be seen also as a sacrifice to atone for his own overwhelming oedipal phantasies— by this I mean an unconscious guilt resulting from the phantasy that he had murdered his father and desired his mother, as was the later part of the story of Oedipus. The raving psychotic patient could be seen, more specifically, to have been excluded because she was truthfully echoing this violent oedipal phantasy. (We will hear more description of the earlier part of the oedipal myth in the next chapter on HIV in South Africa.) Had the mother's marriage to an electrician disturbed her son, reminding him of his father's suicide by electrocution?

The question was then asked whether the psychiatrist might be unconsciously re-enacting this drama with the retrospective suggestion of electrical treatment for her patient. A further shaft of light was suddenly thrown on the story. The case was not just a result of the organic constitution of the patient. The retrospective suggestion of ECT was simultaneously a re-enactment in the hospital of the patient's deep upset over his father's suicide and a means to shut out and ignore the awful oedipal drama. The diagnosis of a situational crisis was also a severe trivialisation of the painful reality of what the patient was going through in his disrupted family life. Did the doctor and the group want to acknowledge the facts of suicide, murder, hatred, revenge, and sacrifice, or to reject them as too painful and distressing? In the end, the group was able to follow and make sense of the reality of the case because of an analytic line of enquiry that began with the comment: "someone is being excluded" (for speaking an unconscious truth). Dr L, in particular, was extremely surprised by the newly apparent truths of the case—an experience that may have helped her to move away from her previously vigorous assertions of psychiatry's organic basis. And, in general, the group had also been given a very effective observation of the mental mechanism of repression—one which they had all experienced in the session through their exclusion of psychological truth in favour of ECT and organic treatments, in the same way as the doctor in her exclusion of the "raving" patient. The importance to the psychiatrists in the group of their clinical enactment—in their wish to prescribe electrical treatment—became a horrible obsession. When noticed, this enabled understanding of the unconscious derivatives resulting from the impact on a son of a father that kills himself in such a way. The unconscious had burst through with the psychotic patient having to be excluded in parallel with the exclusion of the unbearable affect of the case. By eventually accepting and considering this psychic distress, however, the doctors may have learnt the clinical value that being aware of such pain can have for their psychiatry in general.

Case 4: abused and abusing

Dr M presented a case of a twenty-two-year-old single woman whose father had died in the last year or so. She had recently taken an overdose and been referred to a psychiatric outpatient department with a diagnosis of depression. The patient was Catholic and the doctor was shocked to find that his patient had become pregnant for the third time in the last two years. He had realised with some horror that she had conceived around the time of her first appointment with him, when he had decided to see her weekly for about four or five months to help her work through, as he saw it, her grieving reactions. He thought that she was a nice, pretty, diminutive young woman in need of help. However, he also described her as having two states of mind: a poor, innocent young victim, but also a cold, callous, hurtful woman who would not do anything in order to make her life and her doctor's life easier. She had an Asian boyfriend who was several years older. The patient was adamant that he must not know that she was pregnant as he would be upset or even devastated.

The young psychiatrist was feeling quite out of his depth and did not know what to say to his patient. The doctors in the Balint group considered whether the patient would know about contraception, and eventually a view prevailed that she probably did. One participant suggested that if she was aware of contraception then her pregnancy could be thought of as a form of attack. The group was then able to look at the possibility of attack as being an unconscious motif directed towards the boyfriend, the patient herself, and also the doctor. The psychiatrist felt stuck—what should he do? He had said that the patient was attacking herself by taking the overdose—a reaction to her father's death—but whatever he said to her seemed to have no impact. The group was then able to look at the mechanisms of being stuck, as well as of aggression. One doctor speculated further on the idea that the patient might be full of sadism and masochism in response to the recent loss of her father. Some of the woman's history now emerged. She had grown up in a family with a significant lack of emotional stability. If she thought for a moment that there was some stability in her home she was soon made to regret such a feeling. For instance, her mother had recently phoned to say, "Please come home, we need to see each other." When she did visit, she found her mother in a drunken state. She also felt that her father was uncaring and unloving. The patient described what seemed to have been an unhappy, even perverse, family atmosphere.

I suggested that perhaps the patient felt herself to be both abused and also abusing, and that she could be in both states of mind towards herself, her pregnancies, and her doctor. This helped the psychiatrist to understand how she might feel as a victim. He thought that he might be able to rescue her, but he was also able to conceive (note the meaning of the word) that he might become, in the transference, a victim to her. This would apparently mirror the way that the patient's unborn baby (or babies) could be functioning as a device to apparently heal the adult in a deferred messianic manner, never to actually be born. Both she and the baby could be seen as being abused in this dynamic. The serial terminations of the pregnancies could then contain feelings moving unconsciously towards death, a form of repeatedly enacted mourning in connection with her father's death.

The presenting doctor then made the analogy that it was like he had operated on some small lesion and then, to his surprise, found a massive cancer. He felt that his finger was inside the cancer, and he wanted to get out and close the wound up as quickly as possible. His phantasy continued as he described what it might feel like if he removed his finger, such that cancerous stuff would pour out all over him. He felt quite frightened. At this point I said that, as well as the two positions in the psychology of sadomasochism of being victim and abuser, there was a third possibility of being a voyeur. Sometimes the only role for the doctor at a certain moment is to watch and to see and to feel the patient's pain, without being able to suddenly magic it away. At this point the seminar became quiet. One doctor remarked on how difficult a patient with sadomasochistic structures could be. I said that to be a psychiatrist it would help to have a thorough knowledge of such mental mechanisms, but that to do so could also be very painful, as their quietness was indicating. The group became animated, saddened by the pain being revealed and felt by both the presenting psychiatrist and the group. One doctor said that feeling pain was not of much use, and that maybe one should stick to the positive things. Yet for most of the others there was a sense that although knowledge may not necessarily help the patient directly at any particular moment, it does help the doctor to locate what is happening. If we know more about unconscious states of mind, including affect, we might at least feel more stable in experiencing the horrors of some patient's lives.

The doctor who presented the case now seemed to have a much greater awareness, but he still did not know what he should do. Somebody said, "Well you still have three months to look at these issues with her." There was then a debate about whether a doctor should finish treatment at the time originally stated or in some cases continue. The general consensus was that the doctor should not be seduced into continuing to see the patient indefinitely, becoming the "whipping boy" of a patient that keeps bringing sadomasochistic pathology, and having to keep swallowing it. Instead, he had the opportunity to show her an ending that was different from a termination. I then said that he might be able to prepare her for psychotherapy—that if she was able to end treatment with him and perhaps come back in six months' time, without having had another pregnancy, and if she wanted to investigate her mind, she could then be referred to a psychotherapy department. I also warned, however, that it was important to be wary of the phantasy that the psychotherapy department might be able to do magic things with vast cancers. The doctors then had a discussion about outpatient psychotherapy as sometimes being something equivalent to having a heart transplant. In other words, that there needed to be some appreciation—in view of the patient's sense of an unmitigated, awful upbringing—of how large an operation such a psychotherapeutic task would entail. These junior psychiatrists were then able to grasp the unrealistic scale of such a task, and that, as doctors, they could not be expected to cure all patients. Some psychiatric patients might be incurable for a period of time, in the same way that incurability is well recognised in general medicine. Something had begun to be understood. It was not the doctor's task to cure all their patients, but to help them to tolerate their lives.

Case 5: an unconscious self-representation

The first case presented by a new participant in the Balint group is sometimes an unconscious self-representation. Dr N, a young doctor, presented a case soon after beginning his psychiatric training. He was on call and suddenly found that he became alarmed for no apparent reason about a particular patient on his admission ward, fearing for his safety. He rang the ward and was told that all was well. His concern was undiminished, however, so he rushed to find the patient. His anxiety led the nurses to search for the patient, who could not be found. The doctor searched frantically around the ward, discovered the patient hanging in a bathroom, and was in time to cut him down and resuscitate him. This was an impressive example of a sixth sense that some claim to be a vital element for the medical practitioner. His colleagues congratulated the young psychiatrist. They were not able to further process the anxiety of the doctor in his concern for his patient, however, and the case was left.

A few months later, out of the blue, this young doctor hung himself and was also found and resuscitated. What had happened in such a shocking identification of the doctor's mental state with his patient's? The idea of the patient hanging was an experience left inside the doctor which had not been decathected, left available for the doctor to identify with the ill patient. The young psychiatrist had been harbouring his own silent, private life history, unknown until its culmination in mimetically enacting the suicidal behaviour of one of his first cases. And what of his treatment? He was sent to another hospital, this time as patient, and treated by the consultant psychiatrist for manic-depressive illness, with ECT! Again we see the use of this treatment, alongside whatever else it does shutting out the need to understand the actions and feelings of the ill patient, making certain that ablation occurs. The effect on his junior colleagues in the Balint group was profound. There was a sudden sense in the trainees that the sharp demarcation between doctors and patients, healthy and ill, was not so easily available. To compound the story, when a junior colleague visited the ill psychiatrist on the admission ward, he discovered his friend hanging again, made to recreate the original scenario of the doctor discovering and saving his hanging patient.

Doctors are vulnerable. The participants in the group expressed and shared the opinion that the job of being a psychiatrist is at times very, very stressful, and that perhaps mental illness could sometimes be infectious, like a disease. The group was then able to acknowledge the usual defensive strategy of taking sick leave for forty-eight hours, having 'flu ("having flew …"), in order to escape from the mental intensity of the work—rather than to have a breakdown. They were also able to see that a car accident of a psychiatric colleague, for example, may be more than just "one of those things", and may well represent a concealed suicide attempt. In the face of such a terrible enactment by one of their colleagues, many of the doctors began to realise that knowing more about themselves might be a sensible thing to pursue.

Of course, there may be an institutional temptation to give an ill doctor a glowing reference so that they can be transferred to work in a distant part of the country—out of sight, out of mind. Whether it is good for the doctor's patients or for the doctor themselves can be a very hot issue to handle. How do we as trainers bear to face trainees that are unsuitable for psychiatry in terms of their character, in terms of a mental illness, or in terms of the use they want to make of their patients? It is essential to do so. Some people are not suitable for work as a psychiatrist, and it would be helpful for both themselves and their patients to find a way of discussing their illnesses, unsuitable characteristics, or inappropriate motives for pursuing psychiatry—and a way of understanding themselves through their own analytical treatment. Yet the alacrity with which ill psychiatrists are sent away for urgent treatment at another hospital usually precludes any consideration of the impact they have on the rest of the hospital—its patients, doctors, and nurses—and at the same time re-enforcing the culture of a stiff upper lip and defending against the possibility of a psychoanalytic understanding.

Case 6: the party

The group began with the theme of an old professor leaving and a new one arriving. The meeting had been just starting in an anteroom to a lecture hall in which the old professor was finishing a lecture. Everyone leaving the lecture interrupted the meeting by passing through the room, all except the professor. One of the doctors had seen through the door left slightly ajar that the professor, now alone in the lecture hall, was looking at a celebratory picture of himself which had recently been hung on the wall. After some minutes he also passed through the doctors' meeting, interrupting it and talking to one or two people. There was also another theme in the group about parties. The professor was having a leaving party, and there was also a party for a junior psychiatrist who had just left.

One doctor then offered to discuss a certain case, but a colleague exclaimed he must not. A new psychiatrist then arrived at the group. She was initially ignored as the group began to talk about why they were meeting. A joke then followed about how there was going to be a grand college leaving party for the old professor, and that the new one would be meeting the junior psychiatrists for cheese and rolls the following week. With so much discussion of food I commented that the new doctor must have been wondering what she was going to be eating here in the group. There was a desultory silence. I remarked that it had already been mentioned that a clinical case can often help the group out when it is stuck, and that one had been offered, but it seemed that we must not hear about it. There were only twenty minutes to go when Dr O did, in the end, present the case he had previously been dissuaded from discussing. It was concerned with an extremely damaged woman who was a self-mutilator. In the past she had managed to cut both of her ears off, into bits. Then a few days before the meeting, at her birthday party on the ward, she disappeared to the toilet, cut her tongue in half, and flushed it away. Dr P, who had not wanted to hear the case earlier, had been on call as the attending doctor at the ensuing bloody emergency.

There was only a short time to talk about the case, and the psychiatrists wondered about the diagnosis of autism or not. It seemed that the patient's mother was schizophrenic and that the daughter had been brought up completely without concern or care, apparently treated as if she was a cat, and often locked in the attic. Someone suggested that cutting herself was a way of obtaining relief. Another of the doctors suggested that the behaviour was highly sexualised, but the most salient feature was that she seemed very content with what she had done, with blood pouring out of her mouth, smiling and laughing on her return to the ward. Dr P was then invited to say what it had been like to experience the emergency. She said that she did not have any equipment readily available to clamp the tongue. The nurses had held tightly onto gauze. She immediately sent the patient off to the main emergency department at the local hospital. Later, the surgeon rang up, very angrily asking how the patient could have been allowed to do such a thing, and implying that it was the doctor's fault. Another doctor in the group spoke of a new consultant who, within a week of arriving, had to deal with a patient killing herself, and then to attend the inquest on her death. It seemed that there was a fear being expressed in the group of things being out of control, especially when there were new staff around.

As we were very near the end of the seminar, I intervened to observe that we had been talking about parties, and that, beneath the joviality of the parties that linked the patient's birthday and the professor's leaving, there was the shock and horror felt by those of us who were left. It was difficult to adjust to a complicated and horrific case in such a short time, but the telling of it could perhaps make sense of the beginning of our meeting, with the jocularity and celebration of endings. Maybe there was a sense that those colleagues who were having their parties and leaving were making an escape, leaving the rest of us to bear witness to the sadistic material of the patient, for example, forcing everybody on the ward, and now in the Balint group, to look at what she had done. One of the doctors then suggested the important idea that perhaps the professor represented all of us, looking in the mirror to ascertain what price he had paid for staying so long. What parts were missing and what does being a psychiatrist mean in terms of having to face so much trauma? What price do we pay?

The cutting off of a tongue at a birthday party and the horror of the patient's mind projected onto the staff by the smiling attacker had become an unconscious template for seeing the party for the professor as a kind of cannibalistic feast. I am relating this to Freud's ideas of the primitive instinctual wishes of incest, cannibalism, and murder, as described in *The Future of an Illusion* (1927c), and his view of human nature as antisocial, rebellious, and aggressive. The severe trauma resulting from such violence was the "food" of the psychotic patient who attacked the staff and the psychiatrist through a somatic enactment, perhaps the only means at her disposal to demonstrate to them the intense pain of her upbringing. She herself was free of those feelings, having successfully projected them onto the psychiatric ward of staff and patients supposedly celebrating her birthday. She was also unconsciously indicating that, by cutting her tongue, no words would or could be spoken. This act at the patient's birthday party powerfully connected in an unconscious nexus of other celebrations commemorated by the feasting of the psychiatrist's leaving party—jovially covering over the trauma of their professional life with a reminder in that parallel social re-enactment that there is profound psychic pain beneath the surface of staff and patients working together and apart in a mental hospital.

In this vignette, we have witnessed the internal drama of a group of psychiatrists on the receiving end of a horrific assault by a patient. Such trauma is unbearable, yet has to be borne. If the psychiatrist is allowed to cover over such material it may well be left to become part of a pathological structure that the doctor is forced to evacuate, not understanding what is going on in the psychiatric ward and in the mental hospital. Instead, the horror of what patients, and people in general, are capable of doing can be drowned in alcohol, or expiated in the psychiatrist's suicide. This is a serious arena for the future psychiatrist to think about, rather than to brush aside.

Summary

Such demanding work needs a thorough experiential training. During psychiatric training, the doctor who begins to have an internal experience of the unconscious process, and who is in a new position to understand it, will be more able to resist having the capacity for thinking ablated, and better placed to withstand the shock of a trauma projected without mitigation by the psychotic patient. Although the case vignettes have shocking aspects they are just some examples of the ordinary occurrences of severe mental illness in mental hospitals, taking place from week to week. It is gratifying to know that the Balint group is an enshrined part of the education of junior psychiatrists. There are even some groups established for consultants. I have some concern, however, when I hear seminars being called "Balint-type", as I wonder what part of the Balint method is missing from the mix. From the examples offered above we have seen that progress often follows from the simple observation that something has been mentioned but not spoken about, so I have concern for the fate of the groups that are similar but different from the model I have been describing. Finally, it is the patient that leads the psychiatrist in the direction of knowledge by describing their symptoms, myths, and stories in order for them to be elucidated. To do this well, the psychiatrist, as part of the process of being a psychiatrist, needs to know about their own personal history.

CHAPTER FIVE

An experience of a discussion group with HIV medical specialists in South Africa

The blood of many patriots in this country has been shed for demanding treatment in conformity with civilised standards.

—Nelson Mandela, *brief notes in the event of a death sentence* (1964, p. 196)

In this chapter, I will describe a one-day meeting in South Africa in which medical practitioners and hospital paediatricians with extensive experience of working with patients with HIV worked along the lines of a Balint group under my leadership. There were clinical presentations, without notes, and discussions along free-associative lines. The participants did not all know each other. Some worked specifically in township communities, whilst others worked nearby in hospitals. None of the medical participants had worked in a Balint group, but all were interested in working with a foreign psychoanalyst using the methodology.

South Africa is a country overwhelmed by an AIDS epidemic. The annual death toll is huge, and it appeared that there was very little time, and even less resources, for the care of the dying. Medical students, we were told, learnt about hospice care in terms of drugs, but not about the doctor–patient relationship. The dearth of availability of antiretrovirals at the time of the meeting (in the early 2000s) resulted from President Mbeki's view of Western medicine, especially medication for HIV, as a form of colonial plot. Mbeki appointed two controversial American AIDS dissidents—who defied mainstream opinion that AIDS was caused by the HIV virus—to a presidential advisory board on the epidemic. Nelson Mandela publicly rebuked him for his stance on AIDS in South Africa. In such a political atmosphere a cultural phantasy had emerged and become established that medical resources were for the living, and not for those dying.

One of the doctors described how they had had to issue one or two death certificates a day during the previous year, and that this trend had now increased to a minimum of ten death certificates a day. The group discussed a general hardening of the attitude and feelings of the doctor in the face of the epidemic. They were deeply concerned that the medical student of today may grow up with a thick carapace of defence to such states of illness in their patients. Students used to be taught a wide range of general clinical medicine, but now, due to the vastness of the epidemic, they felt concerned that medical teaching was becoming too AIDS-centric. There seemed to be a medical phantasy in the group that the problems were mainly about death, rather than the illness demanding an examination of a wider range of medical and psychosocial problems. Such a phantasy may have been typical of doctors and hospitals across the country.

We were told that, in one particular paediatric HIV unit, seventy-five per cent of the babies born to HIV mothers were free of HIV due to early treatment with antiretrovirals. One could say that this was quite a success story as the majority of those births did not prematurely die. In the particular hospital, however, there was no recognition of this being a medical achievement. Some senior staff in the hospital regarded such good early medical intervention as meaning only that there would be more mouths to feed, and "more of the 'rand cake' being divided up by a larger population".

Clinical vignettes of a Balint group with doctors in South Africa

Case 1: forms of blindness

Dr Q provided an initial and brief vignette. A father, who had since died, had infected his wife and their two grown-up daughters with HIV. The elder daughter, twenty-two, attended the doctor, who diagnosed HIV and offered immediate treatment with antiretroviral medication. The doctor was extremely concerned that the patient was going to lose her sight through the illness if she did not urgently take the prescribed treatment. To Dr Q's surprise and profound dismay her mother refused her adult daughter permission to have the medication. It seemed that her mother was concerned not to let anybody in the community know the tragedy that had happened to the family. She specifically objected to a community nurse visiting the family at their home in the township. Instead, and sometime later, her brother brought her to the clinic at the hospital and allowed his sister to have the treatment. The doctor who presented the case was extremely angry with the mother as it was her delay that resulted in her daughter needlessly becoming blind during that passage of time. This story became a leitmotif of the study day, with the awful idea that someone needed to be blind in order for development to occur. This metaphorical horror of doctors and nurses becoming blind seemed to be overtaking the atmosphere of concern in the hospital.

Case 2: Why spend a rand?

A HIV paediatric specialist consultant presented some case material. She too was angry and upset, reporting to the group that she was generally shunned by her medical colleagues in the large general hospital that she worked in. One of those medical colleagues asked her why money was being wasted on dead and dying children as, in his opinion, the hospital budget could not afford such a paediatric department, especially as "the patients just die". "Why even spend a rand?" he said (a sentence that was repeated throughout the day). Surely, the senior colleague continued, the money could be better spent treating cancer patients, as if this represented a "more worthy" use of scarce resources. The group began to share the presenter's anger. I observed that it seemed that, for many doctors working in South Africa, medicine was presently being understood as about treating patients as long as they had no connection with HIV/AIDS, and that somehow the latter was regarded as a separate matter from the great wave of death throughout the country. The doctors in the group became very animated, saying that, of course, in their training and experience medicine was about treatment, trying to cure, and giving life to the ill. And they seemed angry with me at first when I said that my own experience, with some contrast, was of a medicine that was about birth to death, sometimes helping the patient to die. I was told there was no time for such matters, and certainly no money for it in today's Africa. Another colleague spoke of a senior doctor telling her not to waste time clerking a patient who had arrived in casualty, and that it was just not worth the money, as medical labour, because the patient was going to die imminently. It was harrowing to hear such views, especially from a doctor. This was not some warzone hospital that needed to practise triage. Rather, the impression was given that doctors should stay far away from the newly arrived patient, even just assuming their early death rather than considering that the patient needed to be clinically examined.

* * *

I wondered about a moment's kindness and concern towards a patient, which would not cost a rand. A doctor just being in touch with a person who may have been dying could be very valuable for the patient, who might thus feel cared for. For the doctor also, this could enable feeling for an individual person, in contrast to just another faceless example of the overwhelming tide of AIDS deaths—a tide that can feel like it is threatening to overwhelm the doctor. Giving a kind moment might sustain the doctor, prevent arrogance as a defence against fear, and militate against early burnout in the professional. Such thinking was not part of the defensive cost equation that we had been hearing about, however. It seemed that so many doctors, who did not want to notice a medical connection to death, were living in the blind certainty that they could provide better clinical care as long as HIV was excluded from the work of hospitals, doctors, and nurses. An example of the impact of this on the social systems of hospital life was described above in the material of the medical consultants, in a prejudiced manner deciding to shun the hospital's HIV-specialist paediatrician. Their underlying phantasy seemed to be that the separation of one specialist from the rest of her colleagues would protect the other doctors and the hospital from catching the infectious and deadly illness. Many doctors seemed to be terrified of catching HIV, without realising their pathological anxiety. This would account for their fear of approaching the next black patient collapsed in the emergency unit. In a similar way, in the earlier case about the daughter being allowed to go blind, there seemed to be an avoidance of the possibility of examining how the father's two daughters were infected with HIV—instead, just an assumption that being in that family was sufficient explanation. The possibility that the HIV-infected father had infected his wife and both daughters was left unspoken, as was the possibility of incest. The doctors similarly left unspoken their non-medical phantasy that being present in medical attendance would somehow be the trigger for their susceptibility to catching HIV without sex.

Focusing more closely on the dynamics and phantasies surrounding paediatric care, we can start by observing that the death of babies and children in South Africa is just too commonplace. In Ancient Greek mythology, the myth of Oedipus has King Laius wanting to murder his son, Oedipus, by leaving him to die on the mountainside—the father is frightened of the oracle who implied that his son would kill him. Meanwhile the mother, Jocasta, is faced with the choice of either fighting her husband for her baby's life or colluding with his death urge. Some of the doctors in the hospital seemed to be in a similar state to Laius—unconsciously wanting the death of babies so that the paediatric budget can be given to a more deserving department elsewhere in the hospital. To examine the oedipal dynamics more closely, how does the death of a child help the adult? In the myth, it is an attempt to prevent a father from being killed by his child and also to prevent a mother from being infected by sleeping with her child. Also, the powerful phantasy of killing the child can act as an unconscious antidote to the fear of death in the parents, speaking to the idea that if the child is killed then the parents may survive—a disturbing perversion of the idea that we can transcend mortality by living on through our children.

To return to HIV/AIDS, the birth of a baby infected with HIV seems to be a sign that someone has had bad sex, infected sex, or death sex, and this is seen as shameful, something that must be hidden. Bad sex includes a husband or wife having sex outside of marriage and getting infected with HIV, which is then brought from outside into the centre of family life. The husband often brings death into the marriage, with the potential for murdering the partner. In addition to this, a common protective African myth is that an antidote is to sleep with a virgin, putting daughters at particular risk of being victims of incest and infection. In the oedipal context, the increase of incest in society may also indicate that the baby or child is imagined as innocent of illness—as if the child starts "clean" and is then infected by the adult. And so the passing on of the HIV to the child attacks the child, as well as projecting the violence and death onto them and away from the adult. Being blind to these defensive strategies is a common factor of such perverse solutions, and the murder of children an unconscious solution that needs to be out of sight and out of mind, even to some doctors. This also explains the desire to ignore the dying patient. The doctor's avoidance of the patient, or the mother preventing the doctor seeing her daughter, maintains the thought that the epidemic has nothing to do with the doctor. Blindness has to continue in order to maintain such emotional division. Staying away also means that the unconscious guilt about wishing for the child's death, in order to protect oneself, is also far from insight. For some doctors, then, there is a large unconscious split between life/treatment and death/HIV. Such psychic defences mean that certain doctors avoid patients either known or just imagined to have HIV/death, allowing the doctor to feel that they are protected and better able to cope.

Another implication of this division between life/treatment and death/HIV is that there is an unconscious association of sex with death, rather than with the creative possibility of reproducing life. Sex can lead to babies and life, but, in today's South Africa, sex means being potentially infected with death. Such a change of society's perspective means being blind to:

- kindness and concern to all patients;
- sex as love;
- sex as creativity;
- death as an ordinary and normal part of life.

All of these creative possibilities become ignored by the hardening heart of the doctor who exchanges the death of the baby for the life and medicine of the rest of the community. Such a hardening kills the kindness and love in the doctor, who steadily becomes emotionally dead.

Case 3: Where did it come from?

A fifty-year-old matron in the hospital had asked to meet one of the hospital's consultants, Dr R, as she wanted to be tested for her self-diagnosed illness. Although it was not openly mentioned, Dr R wondered about the possibility of her having contracted HIV. The senior nurse then refused to have the tests that she had at first seemed to desire. Some months later she again requested tests from the doctor. These were completed but the patient then refused to be given the results. In addition, she asked to be referred elsewhere. Dr R had seen the results herself, discovering that the patient was HIV-positive. When she saw the matron she decided, nonetheless, to inform her of the test result. Furthermore, she said that it was unhelpful to not take antiretrovirals at a time of feeling well, as this was an appropriate and effective time to commence the treatment. The doctor later heard that one of the matron's friends, also a nurse, had shouted at her for not taking the medication.

Dr R then began to realise that she had declined to ask her patient about her sexual history. She knew the matron's husband had died a few years before and that the patient did not wish her children to know the truth of his diagnosis, as well as her own. This was despite the patient's considerable clinical knowledge in her position as hospital matron, which included being a role model to her staff—with the particular ideal of being an exemplar of healthiness. The matron's behaviour was another example of a state of blindness, as if it was better to maintain a myth of no sex, linked to a phantasy of no death, than to accept knowledge and take a lifesaving treatment. Whilst prolonging her life, treatment might mean that her children would know her diagnosis—yet it seemed that her children must not know that their mother had a sexual life. Acknowledgement of the equation "sex is death" had to be suppressed in the family, leading to death, and preventing the disclosure and acceptance leading to knowledge and life. Dr R then realised that the reason she had not delved into the patient's sexual history was that such a question might imply that someone was to blame. Did her husband infect her, for example? Where did he get HIV? Or, had she had an affair herself? Did she prick her finger on an infected needle at work? Again, there is a sense of blindness, this time in the reporting physician, attesting to the power of the anxiety surrounding the clinical subject of HIV, and leading to a wiping out of medical perspective.

* * *

It is understandable that the patient and the family fearing the condition of HIV may attempt denial as a mechanism of defence. However, many acts by senior and experienced doctors and nurses reveal a clinical anxiety as deep as if they were dealing with the plague, evoking primitive unconscious defences, despite denial, against catching the plague oneself. The evasion of clinical engagement and the contempt experienced by some patients and staff by doctors is a measure of this profound fear. This is not the usual medical attitude towards patients with tuberculosis, syphilis, or other virulent infectious diseases. And there is no particular dangerousness of the sexual attachment of the HIV virus, as doctors can invariably work competently and safely in such areas by taking simple precautions. Instead, I suggest that the unconscious fear evoked by HIV is due to the scale of its massive assault on family life and society, its vast morbidity suggesting that no one is free from imminent infection and death. As the general practitioner stated at the beginning of the day, he was presently writing ten times the number of death certificates he wrote the previous year. Massive destruction and death without a clear government policy at that time had hugely impacted on the medical profession by evoking blindness as a method of not seeing the unbearable scenes presented to doctors and nurses every day (we could also include the politician here).

As for treatment, all that seems to be available is to see that which is terrible and utilise all medical, social, and political tools to help as much as possible, treating the patient, the staff, and oneself with respect and dignity. The argument is almost persuasive; it has been spoken often. What value is psychoanalysis in South Africa when there is a desperate shortage of food, housing, water, jobs, and education? There is a HIV/AIDS epidemic of 4.2 million carriers of the virus in South Africa (Sidley, 2001, p. 447). The destruction wrought by apartheid over so many decades is now seen in the blasting apart of so many families, and in the perhaps inevitable expression of great social violence. In the pressure cooker of the townships, containing huge numbers of poor black Africans living in cramped, corrugated-iron huts, the violence and the attacks on human rights, and on the dignity of human beings and family life, was huge, as apartheid intended it to be. Children were often brought up without families and with distant fathers, and detached adults lived in marked poverty. There was seething sexuality with massive aggression, and children became an easy and common target for rape. Such traumatic environments do not exist in, say, the UK. Of course, some children and adults in the UK do bear the burden of deep mental and physical scars, but not to the intensity and scale as in South Africa, and much of the rest of that continent. Psychoanalysis may indeed seem an esoteric discipline, and more useful for those who already have the basics of ordinary life. Yet, with all the fear, rage, degradation, lust for life, and creative development evident in South Africa, the discipline of psychoanalysis can be an essential tool with which to think about such forces. As I have demonstrated, acting on phantasies contributes to a deteriorating reality—in one case the metaphorical blindness to that reality resulting in a woman's physical blindness. The chronic nationwide trauma of human rights abuse, etched into the mind, needs all the devices available to develop understanding and to promote change. The mental health worker burdened by the excessive demands of a hugely damaged population can in time become burnt out—made cynical and near dysfunctional from being too long at the edge of the battle. It is at this place that psychodynamic observation of both oneself and the other is valuable, and this is my motivation for reporting on this single workshop as an instance of utilising Balint groups.

PART III

ASSESSMENT

CHAPTER SIX

Why a model of psychodynamic assessment?

To the inhabitants of these arcades we are pointed now and then by the
signs and inscriptions which multiply along the walls within, where
here and there, between the shops, a spiral staircase rises into darkness.
The signs have little in common with the nameplates that hang beside
respectable entryways but are reminiscent of plaques on the cages of zoos,
put there to indicate not so much the dwelling place as the origin and
species of the captive animals.

—Walter Benjamin, *The Arcades Project* (2003, p. 876)

The art and science of psychodynamic assessment is a very complex task. Whilst being a worthwhile subject, the question of how to first examine a potential analysand does not seem to occupy a central position in the now vast range of texts on psychoanalysis. In some ways this is strange, as a patient initially consulting for a psychodynamic opinion on whether it would worth them pursuing analytic or psychotherapeutic treatment has always been at the core of psychoanalysis. Perhaps for classical analysis all patients initially attending were welcomed in the hope and expectation for both analysand and analyst that it would prove efficacious. To begin with, I propose a brief journey through the history of how the concept of assessment was developed.

Freud writes about assessment in his paper "On Psychotherapy" (1905a), and again in "On Beginning the Treatment" (1913c). His views on letting the patient tell their story in their own way, on speaking one's mind, on valuing states of resistance and repression, and on the specific importance at the start of treatment of the issues of time, money, and the use of the couch remain essential and valuable today. As early psychoanalytic thinking was being taken up by some of the psychiatrists in Vienna, Zurich, and Berlin, such as Breuer, Jung, and Abraham, the medical-psychiatric models of assessing patients developed more confidence in ascertaining the potential meanings of symptom formation and affect distortion. It is important to note that, as well as presentations of neurotic and depressive symptoms, patients would present with severe psychopathologies such as psychosis, or what would later be called borderline states, which some patients—realising that the treatments offered in sanatoria were insufficient—brought with hope to the new world of psychoanalysis. Kraepelin first wrote about dementia praecox in 1887 (pp. 21–29); by 1911, Bleuler redefined the syndrome as schizophrenia (or "split mind") and went on to describe its positive and negative symptoms (Bleuler, 1911).

Since that time, there have been important analytic conferences on the topic of assessment. There was a symposium at the New York Psychoanalytic Society on "The Widening Scope of Indications of Psychoanalysis" in 1954, where Leo Stone, Anna Freud, and Edith Jacobson spoke, in which patients with severe character and borderline disorders were considered as potentially treatable. Another early intervention on these matters was *The Clinical Interview* (1955), by Felix Deutsch and William Murphy, an important text of its time, and published in two volumes: *Diagnosis* and *Therapy*. It was written from the perspective of different states of illness with particular emphasis on the psychosomatic, broadening and extending the field of psychoanalytic assessment to include the body. Balint's important text on general practice, *The Doctor, his Patient and the Illness* (1957), went further, taking account of the psychic bonds between doctor and patient, and their great potential for therapeutic efficacy. In 1967, the IPA Copenhagen conference was titled "Indications and Contraindications for Psychoanalysis". The papers concentrated less on categories of analysability and more on the potential use of analysis by the patient. In "The So-Called Good

Hysteric" (1968), delivered in Copenhagen, Elisabeth Rosenberg Zetzel differentiated between treatable and malignant forms of hysteria. This latter paper was a particularly important moment which described a direction in the clinical interview that allowed the assessor to develop a mode of listening to levels of resistance—resistances which, for some patients, might mean that the task of analysis was too fraught with states of aggression, persecution, and fearfulness, and that, despite the patient's apparent desire for analysis, this was clinically contraindicated at that particular time.

Such developments brought a need to assess patients in more psychodynamic depth. It is this new beginning that the present chapter seeks to describe—how the psychodynamic psychiatrist began to observe and be thoughtful about the meanings of symptoms and the psychological development of their patient. Psychoanalysis does not need to be coerced into being an area of medical science or practice. Whilst doctors do need to assess, diagnose, and treat their patients, when faced with the field of the mind and its meanings the diagnostic procedures and tests available to somatic medicine are far less imbued, than psychoanalysis, with the centrality of the position of the doctor as healer. Certainly the notion of a positive transference to the physician has been long known and valued—the patient often in a therapeutically regressed state of mind, as if reverting to being a child listening to the adult doctor, or to a wise parent. Yet this very useful unconscious medical position threatens to unbalance the start of a psychoanalytic discourse in which, in addition to recognising states of regression, it is essential to be sensitive to what such a symptom is attempting to conceal. This use of the doctor was a newly dangerous medical position to occupy, and one that, at the earliest moment in the new subject of psychoanalysis, brought Breuer to quickly move away from the heat of an erotic transference with his patient Anna O. (Bertha Pappenheim), and to precipitously leave his patient (Forrester, 1990, pp. 17–29). Freud, however, recognised the process of the transference occurring when Breuer was summoned to his patient while she was writhing with abdominal cramps. She said, when asked what was wrong, that Dr B's child was coming, causing him to flee, but allowing Freud to grasp the clinical sensitivity of transference impact within the analytic pair. Freud saw this as Breuer's opportunity to have held the transference, yet Breuer let it slip away, in terror. That famous clash between Breuer and Freud held the kernel of the transference difficulties that would subsequently be revealed both in the analytic and in the medical encounter in general. Balint's contribution was to make the link beyond the analytic consulting room and to find it's usefulness within general practice.

Today there are many different routes to obtaining some sort of consultation of disturbances of the mind. Psychiatrists invariably listen to the surface presentation of the patient as a collection of symptoms without linking the material to unconscious process—and without figuring themselves to be playing unconscious roles in the understandings of a transference and countertransference system. Counsellors and psychiatric nurses, having had a relatively brief training, generally tend to tell the patient to cease their negative ruminations and follow a positive course towards life changes. Psychoanalysts and psychoanalytic psychotherapists, meanwhile, are trained in understanding and working with the unconscious, having had their own analyses and a lengthy training, over several years, of seminars and close supervision of two or three patients. In the psychoanalytic assessment, the analyst will usually offer a long initial consultation of up to ninety minutes. This may be followed by a second meeting, to see what the patient made of that first encounter. Based on the knowledge gleaned, work is then done to discuss the possible treatments suitable for that patient—analysis, psychotherapy, or group, marital, or family therapy—and, if not suitable at that time, arrangements made to return the patient to their general practitioner, with some suggestion on how to work with him or her.

Every consultation is unique and the occasion is always new, even if some bear similarities to each other. The problem with treating the described details as a how-to guide, laying out what needs to be assessed, is that it can feel to the patient as if they are being led along a route, rather than bringing themselves to the meeting. In a sense, such a methodological description is an absurdity, as the ways individuals present in speech and in performative enactment are legion. This is the reality of the consultation, one to which the patient will be invited to bring themselves and, in so doing, to allow the specific qualities of their early environment to be revealed. In particular, an outline of the dance of early infant–mother relations may be enacted and perceived in the encounter. However alarming it may be for the prospective patient to be invited to begin wherever they wish—however unpredictable and disorienting for both patient and analyst—this is the whole point of the patient initiating the dialogue. From the first moment, the use of the object that the consultant represents in the consultation is potentially available to the patient. Such a meeting can be frightening and full of anxiety. The art of the assessor, aware of this reality and able to notice the level of tension—allowing it to rise to a certain level, even to some sense of disturbance—is to find a suitable or bearable level for each individual.

Visiting an analyst might seem similar to visiting a surgeon, and so the patient expects to be passive in the hands of the grown-up doctor that knows how to treat their illness—paralleling the child in the presence of the parent who knows, or should know, how to make the pain better. Crucially, this expectation of the patient places the assessor inside the very process she or he is trying to assess. And so, through a replication of the dynamic forces of early beginnings, the analytic interview at the time tries to examine that very set of data of how the child in the adult expects to be treated, on the basis of their perceptions of their infantile and childhood history. The child made to be afraid of the adult will show similar fear in the consultation. Or anxiety may be the fear of being found rather than remaining in the hidden state, albeit with symptom formation. The child who has learnt to live a mental life separately, using splitting mechanisms, will exhibit such a capacity of aloneness, but this will be a far cry from the ability to be alone in the presence of the other (Winnicott, 1958). In this case, such manifestations of alone states of mind are not the indications of a nascent capacity for creatively being with oneself, but are instead reminiscent of early trauma. They are most easily ascertained from the countertransference affects in the assessor, who might feel a sense of distance or lack of engagement. Again, it is worth pointing out the value of getting as much experience of assessments as possible, such that one is able to quickly evaluate the alone-distant presentation, even in the midst of a patient who exhibits a busy life on the surface whilst harbouring a repressed, empty life underneath. This is the subject of recognising the false self.

The point is not to enact such things in a way that causes more anxiety but rather to be in a position to notice such subtle reactions, as they can throw light on the development of early object relations. As such, they are the harbingers of the need to know the patient's history (and of their own curiosity of this history)—that is, the history of their unconscious object-relationship system. Asking too many questions can impede the natural unfolding of psychic material, as it may imply that the patient has to please the other. The natural position of the assessor, as in the psychoanalytic session, is to attempt to be in a neutral place. Then whatever transference and countertransference develop, these can be felt as evidence of the unconscious systems of the patient. Being active in wanting to know and find out is correct in the medical setting, but is contraindicated in the analytic one. Some patients find it extremely difficult that they are not being plied with questions, as their defensive preference would be to adopt passivity in the process. To this dilemma, Balint famously replied, "If you ask questions you will only receive answers", meaning that too many questions on the part of the consulting analyst inevitably produces flat and often defensive answers, leading nowhere.

Similarly, the patient often anticipates what they expect to be asked and factors in answers that are part of their protective shield. It is important to realise that, by presenting for a dynamic assessment, the patient is implying that there is a problem with their character, their history, how they relate to the world, how the world relates to them, their felt capacity to love or hate, or their sexual life. We are being invited into a very vulnerable state beneath the surface carapace. Defences are meant to defend, and the patient, whilst wishing to reveal details about their life, may wish more to prevent (further) pain. A psychodynamic assessment will undoubtedly cause disturbance, but hopefully one that can lead to knowledge and treatment. The reason for not just immediately putting the patient at ease is to determine how they both deal with the silence and their responsibility to reveal themselves, and how they demonstrate their capacity to use the other in the clinical dyad. Here, the intention of a commencing silence presents a valuable underlying matrix with which the patient needs to collide. For some patients, asking a barrage of questions about the assessor and their views—on, say, homosexuality—covers up their anxiety. This is intended to override the present tension of having to deal with the telling of one's story, as well as to anticipate the potential transference atmosphere much later in a treatment. It is a form of protectively running on ahead rather than taking the first steps. Similarly, if the patient resorts to a long silence, it may well be to invite the assessor to ask the questions in a projected defence against that silence. Either way, these are defences against the underlying anxiety around what will happen if they tell their private story and history to another. Not rushing to provide comfort preserves the opportunity to find out something of the patient.

For Thomas Ogden,

> [e]verything the analyst does in the first face-to-face analytic session is intended as an invitation to consider the meaning of his experience. All that has been most obvious to the patient will no longer be treated as self-evident; rather, the familiar is to be wondered about, to be puzzled over, and to be newly created in the analytic setting. The patient's thoughts and feelings, his past and present, have new significance, and therefore the patient himself takes on a form of significance he has never held before.

> (Ogden, 1992, p. 225)

In this evocative paragraph Ogden speaks to a sense of potential creative aliveness that the consultation can provide for both the patient, hearing their mind spoken aloud perhaps for the first time, and a receptive listener—also perhaps the first of such in the patient's life. In order for this to happen, the assessment space must be a flexible place that the patient, perhaps initially surprised at having to initiate the process, may begin to make use of. Thoughts and memories long forgotten can suddenly find a place in the dialogue. One thing can, to considerable surprise, lead to another set of thoughts, showing the patient starting to use the flexibility of the analytic setting. This can lead to new thoughts and to the glimmerings of understandings. It is a form of play that the patient can start to utilise when they have begun to recover from the unexpected beginning, and it often provides evidence that the patient is suitable for an analytic or psychodynamic treatment—not because the assessor says so, but much more because the patient feels that, through this process (free association), things that they say and feel make a sort of sense. Sometimes this can be a flicker of new thought, the unthought known returning from its exile. In such an assessment play-space, the patient—revealing themselves as a character, with a history that forms how they expect the world to treat them in the future—may realise that the assessor, as other, is not fulfilling the part usually allotted to them in such a situation. Having a slight sense that the assessor is not the usual superego imago of their expectations, the patient then feels a glimmer of hope that there can be a different future from the one based on their past. Again, it is another indication that the patient can make use of analytic work. Hope then becomes an important clinical dimension. Its absence can also lead down interesting pathways, towards the questions of when the patient gave up on hope, and why. The argument loops back into the realms of early trauma, where hope is gradually surrendered, or hidden by the protective shield of the false self.

The patient who cannot describe their life and history—which is quite common—has another possibility of communication through enactment, another "royal road" to the unconscious. By this I mean the often tiny activities that can be revealing of unconscious life, representing the unthought, or, to paraphrase Bollas, the unsaid known, when the patient is on the verge of a new articulation. To take a clinical example, a patient arrives for the consultation, unaware that, in pushing open the front gate, they have slightly cut one of their fingers. Despite the patient's shock when they begin to see a little blood, the moment can also indicate something bloody beneath the surface tidiness of the initial presentation. Or it can give rise to a new expectation, that doing something wrong apparently leads not to an expected punishment, or to indifference, but rather to a moment of concern and understanding— a rarity in that patient's life due to the callous nature of their upbringing, which then gradually comes into focus.

The psychodynamics of assessment: the beginning

> It is always dangerous business to stir up the depths of the unconscious mind. This anxiety is regularly misrecognized by therapists early in practice. It is treated as if it were a fear that the patient will leave treatment; in fact the therapist is afraid that the patient will stay.
>
> —Ogden, *The Primitive Edge of Experience* (1989, p. 172)

Why might a person put themselves in the position of visiting a psychoanalyst? The images of the latter in popular perception range from the dangers of entering the lion's cage, with an immense fear of the results, to the banality of a *New Yorker* cartoon in which all things are "amusingly" possible, including the analyst-listener being lulled to sleep. On the one hand the feared encounter with the analyst might tear one to pieces, which includes the possibility that it may be the patient that is the dangerous beast. On the other hand, it might enable, by projective means, a disquieted infant to settle into sleep. The danger is the prospect of a new encounter with both one's own inner world and the internal world of another, stirring up the internal depths. Yet the visit to the analyst is invariably undertaken only when most or all other avenues have been travelled or closed off. Analysis is a possibility of last resort. These days many patients have already trodden the six sessions or so usually prescribed as sufficient by cognitive behavioural therapy (CBT) as an attempt at a cheap, quick-fix solution. CBT initially appears as an acceptable option—certainly one that will not tear the self to pieces. Yet the aftermath of the brief treatment—where there may have been either a great stirring up of conflicts, or else a lid put on further expression or development owing to the short and rigid timeframe—may leave the mind of the patient in a state of added disturbance. There may have been an undercurrent in the therapy of a pervasive positivistic thinking that such a short amount of therapy must "make one better"—only leading to confusion and doubt about whether the complexity of a person's intellectual and emotional constructions can really be understood.

In the analytic consultation, the patient finds that the ordinary discourse of everyday life is left outside the consulting room door and is replaced by a heightened sense of someone listening, in a new and different way. The patient encounters a listening object. The usual discourse in words is listened to with an expectation of many-layered meanings, of metaphor and wordplay heard alongside the rhythm and tonality of the language. Dissonance between the content of the language and its affect is noticed. If unconsciously the patient's expectation was to speak without the other understanding, in the new analytic structure one begins to be heard differently. Yet this very beginning of not expecting to be heard and understood brings with it the problem of the expectation that the analyst has the knowledge to heal. At once we are pitched into the complex subject of the transference. If the analyst misunderstands the heavy burden of being the one with knowledge, then they may be beginning a voyage of power in which the expectation is constantly confirmed that only one of the dyad *knows*—and thus has a special status. For a patient growing up in a family in which the child was constantly treated as being a thoughtless idiot, the ground is quickly and unconsciously laid for a reprise of chronic states of traumatic relating. "Knowing one's place" is then re-evoked with a replication of a passive stance to the clever other. Whilst the analyst clearly has analytic knowledge, they do not have the patient's knowledge of their own particular life. Many patients reify the all-knowing analyst as being superior, as they themselves grasp the undergrowth of inferiority, and this is a matrix around which the ongoing analytic discourse may keep abutting, perpetuating a form of subtle domination by the patient, and an impasse. Yet in the consultation if the analyst does not provide some evidence for the efficacy of the treatment, then why embark on such an arduous and costly journey, in terms of time, money, and emotional strain? The analyst, then, is required to be somehow explicit about the usefulness of analytic treatment, but in an atmosphere that captures a certain authentic modesty in front of the complex task. It is a moment of seduction, often capturing an affective component from early life which will need to be worked through during the treatment that follows. The shape of the patient's impact on the analyst can be appreciated in the beginning of the meeting. How light or heavy the impact of the encounter feels can imply much about how the patient may have been—or have expected to have been—treated by others in the past, the transference beginning its evocations. And why does the new patient attend? Something has gone wrong and is going wrong. This can be in the external world of relationships and/or within the privacy of their mind, with a realisation that the distance between life and their own lived life is diminishing. Aloneness, the prohibition of desires, uncontainable wounds, neurotic symptoms, parapraxes, depression, and compulsions, or feeling more and more lost, are the manifestations of states of illness which in the first analytic encounter may begin to be described. These are some of the things that are breaking into consciousness and creating disturbances. The usual array of defence mechanisms is now unable to contain the thing. Usually for the family, and very often in the psychiatric encounter, such breaks into the present, of angst, violence, and despair, require measures to put them back, beyond, and away from their disturbing effect on others around. For the encounter with the analyst, such disturbance contains the possibility of psychic growth and even healing. But for this to happen, much work is required to decipher the unconscious codes of dream, daydream, and performance (enactment). Presentations of the self to the other in the clinical encounter are often heard in an opposite or alternate register than the more direct and conscious ways of daily life. For instance, the painful affect in a dream may well conceal the fulfilment of a perverse desire. Or tenderness may conceal hostility and aggression, and vice versa. We are entering Freud's discovery of the unconscious, where behind the manifest discourse lie the latent affects and thoughts. As Laurence Kahn recently wrote:

> Between the border that determines the finitude of our knowledge and the "breaches" that pave the way towards the object of our construction, the watchman enforcing eviction is also the gatekeeper that authorizes access. Between the two, the prime smugglers remain free association and evenly suspended attention.

> (Kahn, personal communication, unpublished paper 2013)

The psychodynamic assessment of a patient is a particularly interesting, complex, and arduous clinical process. The general practitioner and the offered visit to a counsellor for a few sessions have not dented the angst, worry, despair, and perhaps emptiness of a complicated life and history. Things have become so overwhelming that the patient has to be brave enough to face telling their story to a stranger. Usually it is very hard to imagine that the analytic listener will understand, rather than be the harbinger of criticism about their life's guilt. The new patient will bring, overtly and covertly, consciously and unconsciously, a great array of difficulties, symptoms, pathologies, complaints, anxieties, and concerns, about relationships, their body, and their mind. In a relatively short space of time, about one-and-a-half hours, some synthesis has to be attempted. Together, some understanding may be found, and the future of the psychic work examined.

There is invariably a tension in the arena of the first consultation between finding out about some of the character, history, and general psychological terrain of the patient, as well as some personal history, yet at the same time creating a thoughtful atmosphere that enables the unfolding of these matters in as light a way as possible. It would be incorrect to understand the beginning as a requirement for the analyst to know about the patient—yet in the emerging discourse, through its details, explanations, omissions, and the atmosphere created by the dyad, the analyst, and also the patient, can notice large, underlying, and sometimes near-imperceptible matters. Through this process the analyst can obtain the knowledge needed to decide if the patient is suitable for dynamic treatment. It is important for the consultant to actively make a decision on the patient's ability to use such treatment, rather than to commence it just because it appears that the patient wants it.

A patient presently unsuitable for psychoanalysis or psychoanalytic psychotherapy still needs help in being referred to a good enough psychiatrist and/or general practitioner. If the patient is very ill but still capable of having psychodynamic treatment, then it may not be possible for a candidate to treat them. Treatment may be provided by the analyst, if they have a vacancy such that the first session of treatment starts the following day—as an expression of taking very seriously the patient's fragile state. Or the direction of the assessment can allow the assessor to refer the patient to a suitable colleague or trainee in good time, in the absence of the necessity of an immediate holding. If the patient is referred to a candidate in analytic training, more focused work is required (as much as may be possible at a beginning) in assessing the patient in the register of mental and physical illness, particularly any suicidal and aggressive tendencies, and the capacity for psychotic functioning. The analyst's experience in having assessed many patients with a wide range of clinical diagnoses enables them to be available with a preconscious sense of what is being conveyed. To use an analogy with painting, the initial sketch may be sufficient, rather than requiring thick, well-defined brushstrokes to manage an early impression. For the patient, feelings about how they are managed in the first meeting can be profound. If it is felt that the analyst is finding out for themselves, this may evoke a memory of childhood affect that one was there for the other, rather than being alone with one's needs.

Yet let us pause. The beginning also means that, whilst the analyst maintains their neutrality, holding to the fact that most of the life and history of the patient is shrouded in mystery, nonetheless some sort of understanding or fragment of clarity needs to emerge for a beginning to be made. Whilst really understanding complex communications built up slowly over long time periods is the work of a dynamic treatment, the assessing analyst, utilising their own experiences of working with a range of different patients, and especially differing psychopathologies, needs to communicate some understanding that captures the patient's imagination. By this I mean communicating enough that the patient may, just, and even against their "better (nihilistic) judgment", feel a little contained or even held—in the primitive sense of a parent holding a baby, rather than leaving the baby to look after itself. Paradoxically, the patient that continues to expect not to be understood at the same time feels a glimmer of hope that someone may be able to hold them—or it, the problem that ails them.

A particular session of analytic work may concentrate on a small area of a person's self, but with the potential for evoking a great canvas of emotions. In the assessment, one attempts to get a feel for the dimensions of this canvas. In the face of such complexity, the interviewer may well feel inclined to ask questions, as the most obvious way of covering the ground. If this is acted upon, the questioner will move around their own areas of interest, ignoring the interviewee's anxiety about what they fear might emerge during the course of the assessment. Where does this leave the patient, who may be made into an inventory of symptoms? Such a consultation might be flat, one-dimensional, and may barely touch the unconscious depth needed for it to be a truly psychodynamic investigation. The more difficult task is for the consultant to let the process unfold, and to let the patient relate to them in their usual manner, without resorting to questions and answers.

As many have noted, Freud himself had no specially formulated interview technique, but made various comments concerning the first interview, such as: "Anyone who hopes to learn the noble game of chess from books will soon discover that only the openings and end-games admit of an exhaustive systematic presentation and that the infinite variety of moves which develop after the opening defy any such description" (Freud, 1913c, p. 123). Freud had the idea of a trial analysis, for some, as a beginning that may develop. Similarly, the consultation can provide a moment in which the patient can experience what analysis really might be like without actually being in treatment. Invariably, as the skeins of complexity and the transference are developed, enough curiosity can be created in the patient to sense the value of continuing the joint project.

Hermann Argelander (1976) pointed out that the analyst has three different sources of data available: objective information, subjective information, and scenic or situational information. He writes, "The reliability of the picture gained of the personality and its psychic disturbances grows with the integration of the information from all three sources" (ibid., p. 28). Scenic evidence includes the scenes conjured up through free association by the patient, alongside the actual atmosphere of being in the scene in the consultation. This is invariably taken in unconsciously by the analyst and processed perhaps as their "gut feeling" or somatic state. In the scenic information, the experience of the situation with all its emotions and representational processes predominates even when the patient is silent. The connection with other data is a secondary act.

The criterion for the reliability of the information is the situational or scenic evidence: "Such information is practically never capable of being checked by repetition, and it is therefore discarded or not mentioned by most interviewers even though it is the richest in what it discloses regarding the prognosis of the therapeutic process" (ibid., p. 28).

Wegner also points out that analysability cannot be understood in quantitative terms measured by objective criteria applied to the patient, and rather that it is measured by the analyst's own subjective possibilities (Wegner, 1992). This is a measure of the assessor's use and valuation of his or her countertransference in relation to the patient. Wegner is also interested in opening scenes, which he describes as the "entirety of the interaction" and which include communications that may be verbal and non-verbal, direct and indirect, along with conscious, preconscious, and unconscious processes of both participants, patient and assessor. In his 1988 empirical study, Wegner found that the opening scene had a significant diagnostic importance, like the relevance of the initial dream.

There is another aspect at the beginning of an assessment that complicates matters further still: the dimension of the institution and its particular needs. A consultant psychoanalyst in the NHS or working on behalf of an analytic training (rather than an analyst seeing patients privately) has to take notice of not just the patient's needs but also to those of the institution. This may mean finding particular types of patients and pathologies for students. Or it may necessitate more detailed assessment in particular psychic areas if the patient is going to be referred to a junior colleague, rather than being taken into one's own practice. The areas of paranoia, schizophrenia, suicidal intentions, capacity for enactment, states of addiction, criminality, and sadomasochistic perversions take on a different slant in a diagnosis when one is assessing patients for inexperienced trainees.

Similarly, in those countries with national insurance it is essential to understand that, beyond the fixed number of sessions that the state will support, the patient will need to be responsible for payment. Otherwise treatment will end with a clerk that knows nothing of the clinical encounter other than that the limit of the state payment has been reached. Having a third party as part of the treatment protocol adds a further level of complexity—in particular, consciously or unconsciously, undermining the confidentiality of the dyad (see the chapter on Analytic Training).

It is also important to factor in whether an institution has to leave a patient on a waiting list or whether that particular person has a more urgent need be seen for the first session, perhaps even the next day following the consultation. This may be vital to some patients with early relationship losses, and failure to act on this may destroy subsequent trust in the wait for therapy some months later. Of course, for others, having their name on a waiting list for a treatment vacancy is apparently very helpful, allowing them to remain in a borderline position of wanting to start as long as they do not actually have to begin—the problem can then erupt just at the moment of being offered treatment, as it destabilises this place of "non-treatment". In a way, one task for the assessor is to function as a ferryman, transporting the patient across to the other side where a particular therapeutic treatment will be available. The journey across to the delivery of treatment may be quicker or slower, depending on any urgency or, conversely, on a sense that the patient is able to wait. Not every assessment finds a need for urgent treatment, but all require either a direction towards a therapy or some explanation of why the present time is not the most suitable.

Earlier I mentioned letting the process unfold. This does not mean that certain areas should not be specifically investigated at a particular moment in that unfolding. A psychodynamic investigation in the consultation involves four specific areas that can show the way in the darkness. These areas touch on the unconscious process and allow depth to be experienced by the patient and the assessor within the borders of that process. These areas are:

- an early memory;
- a dream;
- a masturbatory or sexual phantasy;
- the transference and countertransference in the consultation.

In conjunction with these, it is valuable to gain an impression of the following specific parts of the consultation:

- the first few minutes at the start of the meeting;
- the impact or non-impact of an exploratory interpretation;
- the treatment desire of the patient;
- how the end of the interview is understood and felt emotionally.

This is only one particular scheme, however. It is important to note that, in time, everyone learning such work needs to synthesise some sort of scheme, within their own style. Personal analysis helps greatly in the development of one's clinical ability in assessment, as well as the experience of seeing many patients with a range of difficulties and illnesses. Yet, despite gathering such knowledge over the years, every new encounter still contains the seeds of anxiety for the assessor—resulting from having to bear not knowing what impact the patient will have on them, and what the potential burden might be of their projective systems. Patients reluctantly attend because they have some inkling of the range and power of their emotional unconscious, which, like Pandora's Box, inspires a fear of its uncontrollable destructiveness if opened. Psychoanalysis teaches that an outpouring of such material, as free associations, will in time lead to greater knowledge of the self and an increased sense of one's autonomy. At some moment comes the relief of realising a freedom to know and even speak about the impossible matters that anxiety has hitherto kept concealed, although this is usually unknown to the patient at the start of such a daring journey. Having the guide Virgil alongside him for the journey that Dante makes through the Inferno allows for the possibility of transformation.

Despite providing a particular scheme for an assessment, it is important to realise that it can also act as an exoskeleton for the defence of the assessor if it is pursued too vigorously. The key to understanding this is for the assessor to try to keep their mind free-floating at the same time as listening, hence the value of the assessor having had their own analysis as a means of really discerning the difference between the self and the other. If such a scheme is rigidly adhered to out of anxiety it is likely to provide a rigid assessment. Parts of these excursions into the privacy of the analysand may well need to be suspended in certain areas, but in general the scheme I am describing can act as a useful map for the difficult work of the psychodynamic assessment.

As well as the desire to let the process unfold in the interview, there are facts about the person that it is important to find out—their birthday, particular birth difficulties, and any impact of siblings and deaths, including stillbirths, in the family. Some material about the parents—especially the perceived affect towards each and towards the parents as a couple, as well as how the patient understood the parents' marriage—is valuable as part of the template of the patient's own unconscious object-relational system. Any family history of education, marriage, illness, and hospitalisations is useful. In addition, it is also valuable to know about any suicidal ideas and activities, drug taking, abuse (both mental and physical, such as assaults on the body and sexual attacks), or abortions. If the assessor asks for this network of facts, however, they can create an atmosphere of questions and answers, losing the dynamic edge of the interview. These are matters of much interest in the assessment, and it is better for the patient to speak about their life and history in either an overt or an implicit way as the start of a realisation of the dynamic relevance of the different parts of their life. It is important that the assessor takes notice of that which is not spoken about. For instance, perhaps only one parent is talked about, or there is no mention of a sibling. Such things constitute the unconscious rhythms of the task of what is presented or what is shut off or repressed. Later, the analytic process will connect and reconnect parts of the self that have been dealt with through defensive splitting, or symptom formation, or repression.

In the institution—psychotherapy departments, or analytic societies seeking out patients to be treated by candidates—there is invariably a requirement for the suitability and appropriateness of treatment. Prospective patients are invited to complete a questionnaire about themselves and their life in advance of the assessment interview. Often, this can be a useful device that provides a great deal of information about the person, along with areas from which to commence the interview. However, it is strange for the early impression of the hoped-for meeting to be of a written form, reminiscent of a written exam, and a questionnaire can also feel less confidential than speaking to the ear of the assessor. Their use is not without drawbacks, then, but let us give further consideration to their potential value. The way in which the questionnaire is returned is as interesting as its content. To begin with, it may be returned to the assessor only at the beginning of the interview in an attempt to avoid it being used, or with the expectation that the interviewer reads it there and then, as a defence from real dialogue. Or it may be written at different times in different-coloured inks, pointing to difficulty in answering the questions, but more subtlety to potential representations of splits of the ego. Or a patient might retype the whole questionnaire, making it belong to and come from themselves, the idea of making use of something from another person being too hard to bear. Handwriting too can herald clues, and it can be valuable to consider the difficulty of a person's relationship to others when the letters of the words in their writing do not join up. Obsessional traits can often be performed in the questionnaire when it seems there is not enough space to write everything down, as if this is asked for, the questionnaire then accompanied by several chapters expounding repetitiously on a theme. Paranoid ideation can also very quickly settle on the questionnaire in the form perhaps of disgust that something has to be put down on paper, together with much anxiety about who might read it and whether it will be safe and confidential. While it is reasonable to want assurance of the confidential nature of the assessment, a great anxiety surrounding this can indicate a person's preoccupation with the idea of being found out or hounded. The final paragraph of the questionnaire is also of a particular importance because, after a possibly long read, there can be a sentence hidden towards the end that displays some description of quite profound suicidal intention. This may be to make sure that the questionnaire is actually read, or can suggest a preoccupation with a violence or despair, running beneath the rest of the writing. Alternatively, the fear of suicide may only otherwise emerge at the end of the consultation, when there is little time left to explore its intensity. The early knowledge that a questionnaire can provide can help to avoid this possibility, allowing a vital issue to be brought into the assessment with enough time for it to be examined properly.

The family atmosphere

Whilst maintaining as a philosophy the concern for not asking too many questions, a description of the atmosphere of the family in which the patient was brought up does need to be elicited. The consultation process is considerably more complex than a question and answer programme. Family stories may well emerge in the patient's telling, and this is the best way, but if it is left out of the narrative then it may need to be directly asked about. This can be in terms of an open question about what it was like being brought up in the patient's family atmosphere. This leaves space for the patient to speak about their parents, siblings, or grandparents, and about rows, fighting, loving, or any other feeling, wrapped up in family narratives. Following the patient's lead, and letting the atmosphere of the family sink into oneself, will give an impression of the quality of the important object relationships, qualities of loving, hating, and aggression. Was the parental couple a united body? Was the patient divisive, envious, jealous of siblings? Were there absences or deaths? And what did the patient make of such kaleidoscopic feelings? Out of this matrix and its proximity to the early memory one can build up a notion of the oedipal relationships of the patient, from two-person to three-person relationships and their particular vicissitudes.

CHAPTER SEVEN

The beginning of the assessment

The entirety of the interaction that occurs between analyst and patient, from the personal greeting up to the outset of the interview, including the first spoken sentence ... The "entirety of the interaction" denotes all the verbal and non-verbal actions, all the direct and indirect communications, as well as all the same accompanying conscious, preconscious and unconscious psychic processes of the analyst and the patient.

—Wegner, "Process-orientated psychoanalytical work in initial interviews and the importance of the opening scene" (2014, p. 511)

The handling of the opening of the psychotherapeutic consultation and its initial resistances sets the tone for the whole of what follows.

Before even entering the building, the patient has already had contact with the consultant by way of a phone call or letter, and an appointment time offered. This will inevitably stimulate fantasies of what might happen, together with expectations and hope. The patient has been met at the door and walked to the consulting room. It is important to notice how the patient is dressed, his or her facial expression, and whether a handshake is proffered. One can elicit from the first few seconds a sense of closeness or distance demanded of their relationship to the other. The instant initial effect that the person has on oneself has already made an impression in the mind of the therapist, which can then be compared with the subsequent content of the interview. Someone may step through the door with a smiling bonhomie as if one is just meeting a friend for a drink, and another may shrink as far away as possible from beginning the meeting—one exceedingly anxious patient managed to get lost following me the twenty paces to my own room! The patient enters the quiet space of the consulting room and is invited to sit in a chair and to begin wherever they would like. Once there, one notices how the patient sits, and the general ambience of the patient in the setting of the room. It would be normal for a person to have some level of anxiety about seeing a new doctor for an appointment, particularly one which may well be significant in that person's life. If the person is devoid of anxiety then it is important that this is recognised and considered by the assessor.

Often the patient arrives with quite explicit expectations of what will happen, and may work very hard to have such fantasies realised. For instance, it is very common for the patient to expect to be asked questions by the doctor. After all, this is how other doctors work, and how doctors have treated the person in the past. The patient usually has some standard replies ready in their mind for the questions they are expecting—often consciously, but not always. The idea that they, the patient, should begin to reveal themselves, to talk about themselves and what is on their mind, may well be a unique experience. Although people ask for consultations in order to attempt to speak their mind, this also arouses anxiety, and often intense resistance. It may take a long time before the patient realises who they are speaking to. By this I mean the confusion felt by perhaps being in the room with a primary object, it being unlikely that one would begin to speak easily with or about parents that one may have grown up in fear of.

The patient is confronted with a quiet setting—the room and two chairs—where they and the analyst sit with time and space to try to look at the person's world and difficulties. It seems that some sort of special condition has been established to allow the patient to give expression to themselves. However, this space often arouses resistance in the form of guilt, anger, and hostility. The patient is left to make a beginning, and it is the skill of the therapist to judge the level of anxiety that a person can take in the opening. Given time to begin to speak about themselves, the patient also reveals something of living and being in their system of early object relationships. By this I mean that the way that the patient starts their relationship with the therapist is of great importance in trying to make sense of the patient in their world, and in the context of their relationships past and present. That the assessor does not take control of the beginning, instead leaving space for the patient to manage it, they can be said to be leaving open how the patient may react to them. The corollary to this is that the patient will have a view of how they are being treated, and although the truth might be that they are being offered a setting where they can begin to freely think and feel, this can often be felt as a persecution. It is important that such feelings are exposed in as non-traumatic a way as possible, as they are an indication of how some of the transference may develop if the patient subsequently enters therapy. The assessor can start the consultation by saying something like, "We have time to look at your difficulties—perhaps you can begin where you would like." The patient has now been invited to commence.

Clinical vignettes of the beginning of the assessment

Miss A: aged 30

Miss A's general practitioner referred her for a clinic consultation with the problem that she lacked confidence. In her questionnaire, Miss A wrote that her difficulties had begun early in her life. At eighteen months she was hospitalised with pneumonia. She felt that her father was distant from her in her childhood, and that she received very little physical affection from him. After being later hospitalised at the age of seven with a diagnosis of tuberculosis, she felt rejected by him on returning home. She did not reveal much about her mother except for describing her as "narrow". She married in her late teens, but after a few months her husband left, the marriage unconsummated.

At the consultation this young woman looked rather bland and nondescript. She kept her coat on throughout the interview, although halfway through she did unbutton it. This seemed to be a moment when she began to feel slightly more comfortable. At the beginning she was very anxious, surprised and slightly annoyed that I invited her to begin, and that I did not ask any questions. She began by stating that she had a strict upbringing and difficulty leaving home, and on many occasions returned to live with her parents. Then there followed quite a long pause. After a while I said that I felt there was a likelihood that she might walk out. She eventually and hesitatingly said that she had difficulty in communicating. A little later she said that she felt she might be criticised. I said that maybe she also felt I would be critical of her if she did not communicate. Hesitatingly, she agreed, saying, "Nobody is supposed to have any emotions." It was from this moment in the consultation that she was able to begin to talk. She spoke about her mother usually having "hysterics" when she was depressed, and that her father had no understanding of anything emotional. She feared that in relationships she might be let down from one day to the next. If things were going well, she was always suspicious that something dreadful would happen next.

At this point, from the brief history that I already had, I ventured to clarify her suddenly going into hospital when she was seven. She at once said yes, it was a surprise and, what was more, it actually happened on her seventh birthday, and she was dreadfully upset. I added that it was her second experience at an early age of being in hospital. She said that at eighteen months she had to go to hospital with pneumonia, and that she was diagnosed as having something wrong with her heart. She was not sure what it was, but felt there was a blank, and then said that maybe it was a hole in the heart, or some defect. Her parents had worried that she might die.

The importance of this opening is that the core of her difficulties pointed to her early experience that there was a blank linked to something being wrong with her heart, both physically and, I thought, emotionally. It was this very blank that was experienced during the long pause at the very beginning of the consultation. Of course, I could have asked a multitude of questions at the start that may have covered over the blank that she was unconsciously exposing. Having established that there was a blank, we could then look at its impact on her life and relationships during the rest of the consultation, and find out something about its boundaries. Such material may well have contributed to the blank marriage and its non-consummation. It is also of interest to recall the idea of the French psychoanalysts Pierre Marty and Michel de M'Uzan (1963), who write about a "blank relationship" as a symbolic void in which there is a double deficiency—a symbolic deficiency in the patient and a deficiency of knowledge in the analyst. They coined the term "operational thinking" to describe this process. We will follow the progress of Miss A in the consultation later.

Miss B: aged 30

This patient initially referred herself for a clinic appointment. She wrote very little in the questionnaire. She was being medically investigated for palpitations; she wrote that she was depressed, had difficulty in relating to people, and had not felt like herself for several years; she felt detached and was rarely content; her father died at the age of forty, when she was ten, and she was very close to him. She did not attend her first appointment, saying that she was going on holiday, and was offered another appointment three weeks later.

She was an attractive blonde woman, dressed casually, wearing a red pullover and bright red tennis shoes. Despite colourful attire, her mood was gloomy and she seemed detached most of the time. She seemed to shrivel into the chair, staring down at the floor. Her mood was starkly different from her appearance. She began by saying that she wanted to find out why she did not seem to be able to feel emotion. She felt that she had enormous difficulty with herself and her problems. This included her difficulty in attending her original appointment, leading to a delay of three weeks. She was afraid of the sadness that she felt she might discover. Miss B had been thinking a lot about things recently, and although many thoughts occurred to her she felt that her problem was about other matters. There was then a pause, and eventually I said that her hesitation might be towards looking at sad things with me. She agreed and said she had recently been thinking a lot about her father, and maybe she should begin there. The silence had induced an affect in her that had put her in touch with a potentially central issue of her difficulties, which appeared to be her relationship with her father, his death, and perhaps an impasse in her process of mourning.

By quietly waiting, the patient was able to begin revealing herself. There was a psychodynamic direction being indicated that she had long suppressed mourning the death of her father, perhaps even covered up and compensated for by wearing very colourful clothes, as well as by having problems of the heart (palpitations). In addition, her relationship with her mother seemed to be more in the shadows. The absence of her mother in her presentation of herself became very noticeable, prompting the assessor to take care to not leave the patient's mother out of the conversation later in the assessment. The way that this beginning was managed by the patient revealed a sketch of her unconscious object relationships—resulting in her deep despair about both losing her father and the concomitant absence of her mother. The rest of the consultation could then test this initial hypothesis.

Mr C: aged 50

Mr C was referred to the psychotherapy clinic by his general practitioner with problems of lacking confidence and difficulty in making friends. He apparently wanted to be more confident and outgoing. He did not fill in a questionnaire.

I met a gaunt, anxious, shabbily dressed man who looked his age. Sitting on the edge of his chair, he began by saying that he felt that he might be in the wrong place. He said that he had a phobia and that he wanted a specific treatment for it. Mr C then took out a newspaper article written by a doctor who could treat phobias very quickly without the need of psychoanalysis. He looked as though he was about to leave and asked, could I help him? I replied that it was strange that he was telling me already what his diagnosis was, and asking me whether I could help him when I knew nothing about him. I added that he had to decide whether he wanted to utilise this time to see if we could, together, make sense of his difficulties. He did not seem particularly interested at this stage, but began talking by saying that he was unable to fill in the questionnaire because he thought it had very little to do with his problems. I again commented on the fact that he did not want to tell me anything about himself. He at once revealed the statement: "Well, it's about sex." Then resistance set in, with him saying there was no point in him talking about anything because he had seen a doctor a few years ago, and, "after chatting with him for a few sessions, was suddenly given pills which were no good at all". I said that he was now telling me that he was predicting that I too was going to be useless.

This opening gives some indication of the intense resistance that the patient had towards any mental exploration. It was a sign that I had to proceed very carefully, as his large resistance had been established for a defensive purpose and was protecting him from uncovering a mental state that might well be overwhelming. We will meet Mr C again when we examine his early memory a little later in his consultation.

Miss D: aged 50

Miss D was referred by her general practitioner, who thought of her as being distressed with feelings of being alone in the world. She wrote in the questionnaire that she had difficulty in communicating with others, particularly her mother, who she felt had never let her know that she was loved, instead telling her that she had been unwanted, and only conceived in order to please her husband. She described generally growing up in an atmosphere of feeling unloved.

I met a small, forthright woman who looked younger than her age. Her face was full of smiles as she came out of the lift with a group of people and found her way very easily to where I was waiting for her. Once in my consulting room she began by saying that she was so busy during the day, as well as teaching in the evenings, that she would really not have any time for therapy at all—assuming I thought therapy was necessary, she added as an afterthought. I pointed out that her initial contact with me seemed to be more a way of not talking about any difficulties in her life. In addition, she was signalling to me that her busy life precluded the possibility of any treatment that might help her. She then began to talk in a very vague, shallow, and general way about problems in life and with the world, and how she lived by filling up her external life by being busy. Eventually I said that she was not telling me anything specific about herself. She then said it had taken her a long time to come to the clinic, and she had spent much time composing the form because she wanted it to be done "properly". When I acknowledged that I had read it she talked about how unloved and unwanted she felt herself to be in relation to her mother, but painted her father in glowing terms—that he was her protector, sheltering and teaching her. She described her mother as vindictive, hitting her with a strap, and prying into her life. I observed that her father had not "sheltered" her from her mother, and she immediately burst into tears. At once she tried to push this affect aside as being insignificant, but then did begin to be thoughtful by saying that she had never realised how much she had idealised her father.

This is an example of a patient adopting a torturous and meandering way of communicating as a protective device. I felt I was initially being treated in a very mechanistic way, the patient expecting to arrive, smile, and talk vaguely, and, despite not telling me anything about herself, for me to be able to help her. When her way of communicating was noticed, she immediately free associated on the dilemma with her parents, which appeared to split into a "bad" mother who hated her and an idealised father who loved her. It was when I brought her parents together—in a single sentence—that I was able to give a communication to her that made contact, causing her to feel a real affect. I think this was achieved by carefully noting the absence of real communication that she filled the space with during the opening, and by inviting her to notice this as well. I also want to point out that by making an interpretation and seeing its impact it became clear that the patient, despite the initial presentation of having no availability for dynamic work, was in fact able to make use of such treatment.

Mrs E: aged 41

Mrs E was referred by her general practitioner with a diagnosis of an alcohol problem. She cancelled her first appointment and then demanded an evening appointment, as she was working during the day. She was offered an appointment two weeks later at the same time as the first.

On arrival she began by saying that she felt better since being referred, and felt more in control of her alcohol, but in the last few days had been less sure. She then wanted to know why we were meeting, as well as wanting an exposition on the treatment facilities. I said that I did not know what was suitable for her at the present time and that was the reason for our meeting together for a consultation. Again we see an attempt by the patient to get the assessor to do the talking, as a means of avoiding presenting themselves to the other.

She then said that she did not know what times she could attend, and that she taught until late in the evening so it would be very difficult for her to attend. And anyway, she had no money. At the end of another paragraph about her state of resistance she gave me a smile. I replied that she was talking as if we already knew about her problems and that it seemed that we only needed to discuss the formalities of how she was going to have or be able to have treatment. I added that it seemed she wanted to avoid looking at any of her difficulties, as well as describing her drinking habit, and she agreed. It was very important to highlight this intense resistance and ambivalence towards looking at any part of herself, and to have it acknowledged by the patient at the beginning. She was trying to block the possibility of any understanding of her.

The opening space had been filled with how she preferred not to look at herself. Speaking about such resistance at the beginning of the interview enabled plenty of time to try to find out more, to understand and connect, if possible, with the patient, rather than this being left to the last few minutes of the consultation. Whilst there was not yet an understanding of the reason for Mrs D's position, at least the clinical dilemma was whether she might take responsibility for herself. The consultation actually continued in a similar vein, however, it becoming clear that she did not wish for any treatment other than to perhaps continue treating herself with alcohol. Perhaps her doctor had felt similarly to her, that he was unable to be of use, hence the referral. We will see later the impact of her early memory.

Miss F: aged 35

A woman aged thirty-five was referred with a brief note from her general practitioner saying that she had "sexual problems", the details of which he did not specify. In the questionnaire she wrote that she was "credulous" and generally unforthcoming about herself. She also wrote that her father had died when she was twelve.

She looked younger than her age, dressed in a T-shirt, jeans, and plimsolls. She was attractive and had a smiling, open face, and wore no makeup. Having ascertained that I had read the questionnaire, she was quite shocked that I was not commencing the interview, and at once burst into tears. She asked if I could help, and I quoted something that she had written on her questionnaire: "given the opportunity I always do the consultation of the other person". Through her tears she smiled at this, and, despite not knowing where to begin, started to talk. She said how surprised she was not to have seen her father again and that she thought this had a lot to do with her difficulties, although she did not know how it connected with other things. The patient had started off with a smiling, cheery façade, expecting to do the interviewing herself—her usual method of control. In the totally new situation of the consultation, though, she felt shocked and burst into tears, although I also felt that this was a device to provoke me to rescue her. When she realised that I was not going to do such a thing, she was able to begin talking about her father and her feelings of loss, which were perhaps the crux of her emotional difficulties. Her usual way of managing other people by taking control of the interview may have been an indication of a false self, developed in order to conceal the depressed part of herself. What was particularly interesting was the almost instantaneous way that she tried to initially make contact in a defensive manner, indicating the importance for her of being able to control the object—in a way that she had not been able to regarding the death of her father. The start of the consultation brought her defensive habit of control to the surface at once, and facing that dynamic enabled us to work more on understanding how she functioned in that way in her life generally. Later, we will find out about her dream.

* * *

These vignettes demonstrate the value of being sensitive to how the first few minutes of the consultation affect the patient. For many patients there is a familiar pull towards not speaking about themselves or their difficulties, or even their life in general. Rather, a defensive position is readily adopted in which the consultant is invited to speak as if much is already known about the patient, despite their silence. It is as if it is futile for the patient to reveal anything, a well-known and well-used character defence; yet it is these defensive structures that can present difficulty in life. It seems that an internal state of mind demands that the patient remains isolated and alone, treating themselves with mind-numbing drugs, perhaps, or with alcohol. For some, this is a way to remain in a state of unmourning towards a dead parent, or towards another loss. Such defences of aloneness are *après coup* states of mind that can often be reminiscences, such as the child having to bear to suffer alone in a family atmosphere that did not properly care for them during their early life and adolescent development. If interpreted during the consultation, the early appearance of descriptions that evoke such mental constructions can allow space for the dyad to bring back to life such evocative pictures of the unthought known, instead of them remaining behind a defensive screen of a fixed, unemotional, flat life.

CHAPTER EIGHT

An early memory

Footfalls echo in the memory
Down the passage which we did not take
Towards the door we never opened.

—T. S. Eliot, "*Burnt Norton*" (1936, p. 13)

In this next section I want to develop the idea of the importance and value of trying to reach, during the consultation, an understanding of the patient's early memory. We will follow the clinical material of patients A, C, and E from the previous section.

The earliest memory that the patient can recall is an indispensable part of the structure of the psychodynamic interview. Earliest memories are absolutely specific, distinctive, and characteristic in each person. They can reveal a specific core of a psychic life, the formation of the neurosis, the early object relationships, and emotional colouring, although for all of this a detailed analysis over a long period is required, revealing the myriad of unconscious linkages. The early memory shares the same psychic font as the dream, and is built from the same unconscious processes. It may be the truth or a distortion, but its importance lies in it being a particular remembered psychic reality. Whether it is real remembrance or phantasy is therefore subordinate, a lesser issue in a theory of dynamic consultation. Still, false memory syndrome can be a particular and very complicated factor, and there is a strong need to know much more about this subject in the context of the rest of the consultation. Some patients will attend a consultation with a conscious idea that they have been abused in childhood as a cover for further examination of the rest of their life, history, and symptoms.

Reports of the beginning of memory traces usually describe experiences had around the age of three, although a few slight fragmentary images may be remembered from even earlier times. Terr (1988) found that children suffering early trauma when aged between twenty-eight to thirty-six months could be differentiated from those children who could verbalise their past experiences, as they could do so only in part, or not at all. Of course the internalisation of the traumatic process itself may affect the apparatus of the laying down of memory storage (there is further discussion of this in Sklar, 2011). Fragments of certain early perceptual experiences may occasionally be recoverable in the course of analysis—parental objects such as the sight of the face and the breast of the mother, the smiling or angry expression, the pleasing or disagreeable character of the voice, the soft touch or rough handling, the sight of the hands. More continuous memory begins at different ages in different individuals, but usually not much before the age of four or five. Some people attest to remembering nothing prior to a much later age, for example not even fragments until the age of nine or ten. This is indicative of much repression that the early years are under, and one needs to be thoughtful about repressed states of early trauma of one sort or another. Other people seem to be in touch with a firm memory as early as the age of two.

The early memory in the consultation, like the dream, is another royal road to the unconscious. It is perhaps more fixed than the discussion of the dream, as it is less liable to be influenced by the day's residues. The dream in the consultation can, in part, be used to check the patient's anticipations and hopes, along with the dynamic forces and transference. The early memory has a greater constancy, however, and can act as a window that opens onto the early etchings of life held in the memory store. It is a piece of the person's mental life that has been known for a very long time, although more often lost or in the shadows. Most people when asked for an early memory, and when they remember it, are not that surprised at what comes to mind, as an example of the unthought known. It is something of which they have been conscious at various times in their lives, although its recollection, in the context of the consultation, may sometimes be quite startling.

The early memory is often a tersely sketched scene. In this scene there will be a description in which the early life and object relationship of the person are indelibly printed. It is important to notice the characters sketched in the early memory and their relationship to one another (yet another example of the psychic idea of who is doing what, for whom, and for what reason). The negative of this scene is also of the utmost interest—for example, who might be missing or absent. Is one parent favoured over the other, or a sibling? Are the relationships in an atmosphere of love or hate, activity or passivity, sadism or masochism? What is the affect associated with the memory? If there are no feelings associated with this early memory, can such a thing be understood and felt by the patient? Are there associations to the early memory and where, if anywhere, might they lead? Some patients immediately want to change the subject and wish to tell us another "much more interesting memory". This might indicate that there is something sensitive in the first memory that has been disturbed, provoking an immediate resistance. Some people may, instead of an early memory of a space, or of a drama on the stage, remember a very strong sensation such as a taste or a smell. One person's early memory was of a strange yet distinct and familiar sensation of the smell, taste, feel, and experience of rubber. Could this be a direct representation of a rubber teat on a feeding bottle? The remembered sensation was even more specific, of the experience of warm rubber. At seven months this person was changed from breast to bottle feeding, so the early memory may contain a vitally important latent remembrance of the atmosphere of separation from the mother.

Often a person will spontaneously remember an early memory and will be in contact with an unconscious realisation of its usefulness in the consultation. It can then be taken as a mark of psychic awareness and curiosity when judging the capacity of that person to undertake an analysis or dynamic therapy. It is interesting to consider what the right moment is to ask for an early memory. It is my impression that it is useful to see if an early memory can be found following on from the patient showing some affect in their discourse, especially at the point of being in touch with aspects of their childhood. Once the memory has been described it is valuable to invite the patient to give their ideas about the described scene, including any associative feelings and any connections with their present life and difficulties. The very proposition invites an oscillation between then and now, and unconsciously indicates the matrix of connections and fluidity available in dynamic therapy. For the patient who has very little sense that their past matters, or is significantly linked to their present life, this can be a harbinger of insight. It is important to note that the finding of early memories in psychoanalysis, and their value in treatment, is very complex. In particular, traumatic memories may be discovered after having been sequestered or encapsulated. Therefore, their hidden location, until they emerge into analytic treatment, means that they may not have been subject to psychic transformations and *après coup*, indicating a splitting of the unconscious ego, from which they are disconnected. In such splitting, I am referring to an inability to find a traumatic trace in the phantasy life of both day and night dreams—or in symptoms. Some deeply painful and perplexing fragments have been repressed, made distant in both time and space, in the way that someone can be "spaced out" or mindless in time. It is less likely that such fragments of profoundly dissociative memory will emerge in an assessment, but it is possible, due to the unusual qualities of the atmosphere of quiet listening. Either way, the ability to notice a sense of absence in the coherence in the stories of the past, as they are told, can give a clue to the depth of repression. If the assessor notices this kind of absence, they should realise that treatment will be less effective, or will be ineffective, if the patient is seen with big gaps between sessions. A more intense analytic treatment can be necessary for the absences and gaps that signal deep repression and splitting of the ego to have a possibility for being held and noticed in therapy. The assessor can now continue the consultation with such ideas held in their mind as they search to ascertain the patient's present suitability for psychodynamic treatment.

Clinical vignettes of the early memory

Miss A: aged 30

We met Miss A in the previous chapter when she unconsciously performed in the first few minutes of the assessment the emptiness she felt at her core. She had experienced feeling alone in the world after her mother had told her that she had been conceived only to please her husband. Just after I felt that I had made a real contact with her—following my observation that it seemed that her father, whom she had idealised, had not protected her from her, as she saw it, attacking mother—this seemed like a good time to ask for an early memory. This gave an opportunity to further establish the shown affect, to possibly reveal its historical development, and to test the hypothesis so far. Her early memory was of being on holiday with her parents and walking between them. Her next thought about this was that "of course, it was lovely". I commented on her use of "of course" and she replied that she felt that there had been something quite sinister around and it was dark. She said she did not want to discuss it because they were only thoughts. She could not know if it was real or not. At this point she seemed to be attacking her memory and thoughts as not being trustworthy. It appeared that she preferred to rely on external things. She wanted my support in this to help her get away from "the shadow of her life", of her sense of coming between her parents.

I examined this material by saying that she seemed to be discounting any possibility that she might make some sense of her "thoughts" and feelings. I said that such things did have a bearing on her life (looking back, I may have unconsciously chosen the word "bearing" for its association with childbirth). She was then able to acknowledge that this early memory did reveal how she felt her life had been growing up in her family, under a shadow or feeling that she was living in the dark. It seemed she had unconsciously sketched a "lovely" surface with a sinister and darker picture underneath—of feeling unwanted as a baby.

Her early memory had also clarified a strange remark she had written in the questionnaire, that when attending college she felt herself to have been "between the small fry and the top brass"—surely this could be another way of expressing living between her mother and father in the dark, or how small she still felt herself to be. This is a good example of the ubiquity of the free association that the early memory may clarify, and how psychic truth is inevitably interwoven into many areas of a person's life—although often in too subtle a way for it to be immediately recognised. This dynamic permeated the patient's intellectual strivings, her relationships with others, and her difficulties in sexuality, in which she struggled "in the middle". It also contained a sense of her still living a life as "small fry" rather than as an adult—a subject that one might imagine would be an important part of the matrix of the transference during an ensuing treatment.

Mr C: aged 50

Mr C had said he did not want an analysis within the first minute of commencing. He then quickly jumped from diagnosing himself as phobic to revealing to me that he considered his problems were all about sex. His shabby clothes and demeanour, providing a vivid impression of great personal neglect, made me thoughtful that this man was perhaps very ill. His leap from his self-diagnosis of phobia to attesting to a centrality of sexual difficulties made me aware that his strange verbal connections might point to his functioning at a psychotic level. I had to decide early on whether to accept his lack of desire for analytic treatment in order to avoid opening up what seemed to be a great amount of mental dysfunction, or whether to try and explain to him dynamically the difficulties he suffered and that he would need to endure if he wanted to have a talking therapy. His apparent decision to decline therapy whilst still attending the consultation may have been a defensive ploy—if he expected, as usual, not to be understood. If some real contact was made and he felt understood then the consultation might be of some future use to him. It may, in addition, provide the beginnings of a bulwark against the feeling of being totally isolated in the world. He went on to talk about how he did not have much hope following several previous treatments, and how he had felt the same sense of hopelessness as he travelled to the appointment to see me. It was at this point in the consultation, whilst he was in touch with a sense of pessimism, that I asked for an early memory. His memory was of being in kindergarten. He remembered watching one boy throwing sand into another boy's face. After a silence, I wondered if there was a part of him that was also watching in this consultation—watching and expecting me to throw sand in his face, rather than to help him. He looked at me, smiled, and agreed. This moment of transference was the point at which he was most animated, and the most contact between us during the consultation.

According to his doctor's referral letter he had an older sister and two younger brothers, all of whom were successful in life. When he was ten he had an undescended testicle removed. One year before the consultation he had an operation to fit a testicular prosthesis. The early memory perhaps contained his feelings of being the victim in his family, intellectually, bodily, and sexually. The dynamic of his early memory, however, was for him to be the watcher. This could be understood in an opposite way to my interpretation, his memory being his way of throwing sand in my face to prevent me from reaching him, the victim turning himself into the potential despoiler of any psychological treatment through identification with the aggressor. The victim does this in a state of psychotic functioning, far removed from any thoughts about the impact on his childhood and adolescence, for example, of having to know that he had one testicle.

Mr C seemed paranoid and the early memory could also indicate this, the watcher being projected onto the world that then becomes the bad, feared object that will attack him. His early memory communicated what he expected of the world, as if it would invariably be a sand fight. He was no longer engaging much in life, but had moved to a seemingly safer psychic retreat from which he could watch rather than participate. This had left him unable to get involved in the reality of his daily life as he felt too vulnerable and damaged, needing to protecting himself. We both agreed that this did not seem a suitable time for him to embark on dynamic therapy, but he was able to leave with some understanding of how he continuously protected himself from expectations of being humiliated, and that the surgical removal of the undescended testicle was key to his knowledge that, really, his illness was "all about sex". He departed with seemingly less need for his usual paranoid shield.

Mrs E: aged 41

The early memory of the alcoholic woman, discussed earlier, was of going to London with her mother, and that bombs were dropping from an air raid. She remembered being excited and that she was given orange juice, but she thought not by her mother. When she returned to the country the garage doors banged like bombs going off. This material could have been thought of as containing a screen memory of the primal scene, especially as her sister was born eighteen months after herself. Or it could be seen to have contained derivatives of the anal stage of development, with the description of the bombs dropping. However, this did not seem to be the appropriate level of working in the consultation, especially as she was quite a recalcitrant patient who was nowhere near having such interest in her material. Such a widening of the frame of the material would be more appropriate to the middle of a treatment, and as such was far beyond the present diagnostic task. Instead, I made reference to her affect, saying that her early memory made me wonder whether dangerous things excited her as a general principle in life. She agreed, and also thought this might well apply to her alcohol consumption. With her early memory, the patient had unconsciously revealed a deadly excitement, and, at this moment in the consultation, it was more valuable to be in touch with this affect than anything else.

Mrs E went on to say that when very young she had been left by her mother for a long period in the care of her maternal grandmother. The bombs in the early memory could have been an expression of how she had felt dropped by her mother. The explosive danger of a dropping bomb is then connected with the affect of losing her mother. The memory may also have contained a phantasy of revenge on her mother, and perhaps also her youngest sibling, the patient assuming the position of the bomb itself. Was depression turned into excitement for this patient? Perhaps the orange juice in the early memory, not given to her by her mother, is transformed into another drink, alcohol, in identification with her alcoholic father? Material from an early memory can spark many quiet hypotheses in the analyst. In this case the memory followed on from a dull, resistant beginning of the assessment, indicating that, despite the initial state of stark resistance, there was an unconscious desire to provide psychic material that could start to be understood. This would be an example of an unconscious pull to reveal. It also suggests the hope that can be created by a communication involving free association, and by the insight of a creative linking of past and present.

* * *

Some patients wonder whether any early memory will do, or if it has to be the earliest. Following the concept of free association, it is the earliest memory that comes to mind that is required. Reliance is put on the unconscious positive direction of the patient that desires to participate in a deep communication, and to be helped. Such patients can be contrasted with those that deny any contact with their past. The analyst can sometimes hear the extraordinary idea that the person has no memories at all until after eighteen years, childhood and adolescence under an intense repression. Even when challenged there might be no memory retained at all, such that the defensive system remains intact. This indicates an enormous level of repression of emotional life that so much of a person's object-relational system is removed from conscious awareness. This level of repression suggests that they might have great difficulty in accepting psychotherapeutic treatment, despite apparently wanting it.

If the early memory is asked for because of a lull in the consultation, to fill up the silence, then it may be less valuable and have less impact. I feel that it should be asked for following the beginning of some emotional contact that the interviewer feels in her or his countertransference. If the patient is struggling with an idea or an affect, approaching yet still distant from it, this may be both an interesting and appropriate time to ask. The assessor will at times act as the midwife, unless the patient finds from their own resources a capacity to speak the unexpected associative line of thought. One is leaving it to the unconscious processes of the patient to be more consciously in touch at this moment, or to not. Like so many things in psychoanalytic therapeutics, this is yet another area in which experience plays a large role. It is the countertransference feeling in the assessor that often suggests entering the field of the early memory.

Lastly, I want to draw attention to the way a person may comply with a request for an early memory. A patient who can freely describe the imagery of early memories will be able to make use of a psychotherapeutic treatment in which free association and saying what comes to mind is of great importance. Other patients may ruminate on the request and ponder, as is the obsessional character, if this or that memory came first, without revealing of what the memories consist. Or some will be concerned with totally satisfying the request, which, in their mind, becomes the demand that it must be the very earliest memory and nothing else will do. Here, one can use the process of the reaction diagnostically, as it can reveal the defensive demand of obsessional thinking. This is another form of examining the patient, through their use of an object (Winnicott, 1971, p. 101).

CHAPTER NINE

The dream in the assessment

The interpretation of dreams is the royal road to a knowledge of the unconscious activities of the mind.

—Sigmund Freud, *The Interpretation of Dreams* (1900a, p. 608)

Whenever I began to have doubts of the correctness of my wavering conclusions, the successful transformation of a senseless and muddled dream into a logical and intelligible mental process in the dreamer would renew my confidence of being on the right track.

—Sigmund Freud, *Revision of the Theory of Dreams* (1933a, p. 7)

The sense of conviction that dream interpretation can provide about the reality of unconscious mental activity is unequalled by any other clinical experience. The dream can reveal, with unusual clarity, various aspects of unconscious life, from the etchings of early life and internal object relationships, as memory traces, to memory residues from the previous day. It can provide access to dynamic data with relevance and importance to the clinical interview. The dream can also provide an excellent vehicle to discover potential aspects of transference in the consultation. Whilst it is true that it usually takes

167

a sustained period of analysis for transference to the analyst to settle in its clinical groove, nonetheless an aspect of transference, concerning the imagined encounter, is often present and available in the consultation. Being able to notice such an imagined fragment may well provide an early perception of how the transference will emerge in the fullness of an analytic treatment. Such fragments can indicate the patient's fears of seeing a psychiatrist or an analyst for the first time—fears of madness or anxiety about whether help is really possible, or whether they are irreparably damaged. Many of these imaginings lie on the surface of the patient's mind and are sometimes discussed in a superficial way that avoids any impact of such feelings or belief. This can point to a problem of rationalisation, a defence from experiencing the impact of the meaning and feeling of affect, instead speaking about it from an emotional distance. If psychic authenticity can be discovered in the dream, though, then it has an emotional impact on the patient that is usually inescapable. This leads to a greater contact with any lost or repressed affect and can provide the patient with a greater sense of the usefulness of analytic curiosity. It also begins to establish the idea that one's imaginative apperceptions are valuable and can be taken seriously as a means to further knowledge of underlying levels of the self.

The dream is closely linked to childhood memories as both use essentially pictorial representation. Freud drew attention to the notion that primitive mentation takes place in pictures and can be closer to unconscious process than later verbal representation. Things that are heard and seen in childhood can be turned into pictures in the form of screen memories. Any hypothesis drawn from the early memory about the life of the child still active in the adult can be further tested with the discussion and associations of the dream. If partially understood, the dream can supply links to the dynamics of the past, as well as the present, lived life of the patient. It is an area of the interview in which one may be able to judge whether the patient has a desire and capacity to be in touch with their inner world. A patient with no readily available dream can be partially seen as unconsciously resisting investigation of the unconscious. However, as will be seen later in some of the examples, even exposing such defensiveness can lead the patient to a realisation of this psychic position, and to both a concomitant freeing of associative links and an increasing interest in the process of the assessment.

I have sensed that it is best to ask about a dream during a period in the consultation where there is an expectancy by the patient and/or the analyst that something should or might or may need to happen to clarify the present point of the consultation. In a state of mind where there is an approach towards a vital dynamic or affect or buried emotional content, the dream can facilitate the process of discovery. It is important to invite the patient's associations to the dream rather than for the interviewer to jump to their own. This is to invite the patient to start thinking about their inner world, and this may be a startling, new, and valuable experience.

A clinical vignette of the dream

Miss A: aged 30

The patient described having many dreams, often of being chased by a fire or flood, with the water coming after her. Recently, Miss A had dreamt that she was chasing after a rabbit and then was squashing it to death. She did not appear to have any affect or anxiety about vocalising such a violent thought. Despite having written in the questionnaire that she felt depressed, she had not yet given any indication of such affect in the consultation. I decided to examine this material in terms of her being the victim rather than expressing a murderous rage of her own. I ventured to say that perhaps she feared being drowned, even being drowned in her own tears of sadness, as represented by the water coming after her. At once she began to look extremely sad and started crying, nodding in agreement. There was probably a great deal of emotional life within the web of these dream fragments—certainly a contrast to the blank that we had established in the opening few minutes of the consultation. I made further use of the dream by noting the patient's lack of emotionality in conjunction with violence and murder, and yet worryingly, at the same time, that the dream seemed to chase after her. As fire is a reversal of water this suggested that the dream might have been concealing a repressed flood of tears and depression, as well as pointing towards a similarly repressed fiery anger.

In this example, the dream evoked an outline of a concealed emotional life—a significant discovery for the patient who felt herself to be somewhat emotionless. The dream that was spoken, heard, and taken seriously became a vehicle for the patient to begin understanding that her unconscious life contained the lost emotional traces that she sought whilst simultaneously denying. The very act of describing a dream is one that necessitates an acceptance that the dream is a serious component of one's mental life—and an acceptance that, by looking at a manifestation of unconscious process which contains both day residues and earlier etchings, the dream indicates the nature and value of analytic thinking. This in itself is a rather new form of discourse for most patients. I did not ascertain the meaning of the rabbit, nor much about the killing. This would be a subject to elucidate if therapy subsequently occurred. In the situation of the consultation, one could understand part of the dream in terms of a secretive, sad, perhaps lively part of her self being squashed and killed by another aspect of that self which had been split off. This began to make sense of the blank that had been found, and suggested that she was in a position to accept some responsibility for her history, as well as for her defensive structure. Most significantly, by concentrating on this part of her dream, we could discover the very real, sad part of herself that was usually hidden from both the world and, to a large extent, herself. Although the patient superficially and intellectually knew that she was depressed, this was just a word applied to cover a blank feeling rather than a real acknowledgement of such an affect state. The dream enabled the patient to be brought to an awareness of the power of the unconscious process and the value of the psychodynamic approach, and it allowed a consultative alliance to be formed that could develop the positive transference towards an acceptance of treatment.

Clinical vignettes of dreams about difficulty communicating

Miss F: aged 35—a dream that pointed to unresolved mourning

This young woman, who we met earlier, had been referred with unspecified sexual problems. Her father had died when she was a child. She had dreamt the previous night, prior to the consultation, of looking at a flat with her boyfriend. She was checking that the blinds over a cupboard were down and that the rooms were all tidy. I said that I wondered if she wanted to keep covering things up with a blind (as in being blind) as she had indicated she had been doing for most of her life. She was initially resentful at my remark, and said that she had needed to cover up something very ugly in the cupboard. "Anyway," she said, "everyone has cupboard doors which they keep closed." At once she realised that she was talking about her mind and her body, and smiled with embarrassment. She then became more freely able to use the metaphor of the shut cupboard, and began to speak of her fear that whatever it was that she was concealing inside herself might get out of control, including her sexual life. Here the shut door could have alluded to a shut vagina and sexual life. Yet we could look at this material in another vertex, the closed cupboard possibly also being a description of the early death of her father—something "ugly" and unmourned at the back of the cupboard, interfering with her adult sexual life. This anxiety might have included the impact of letting another man into her life, other than an idealised father—if another man was to get inside her cupboard he might find a dead father concealed at the back.

The dream brought into view aspects of the way that she had closed her mind to mourning the loss of her father, and the intimate and disruptive connection of this with her sexual life. Difficulties in her sexual life could then be gradually understood as a potential interplay between sex and death, a place to begin overtly mourning her father's death. This understanding would enable a focus on her unconscious sense of guilt about wishing for the death of her father. Unconsciously, she feared allowing her boyfriend to be close in case he too would meet an early death. Miss F was able to acknowledge that such matters pivoted around her dream, and so, rather than somebody telling her an answer she could easily disavow in a maintenance of her blindness, the dream gave her space to consider these vital things.

Mr G: aged 60—a patient with torticollis who never dreamt

I was informed by the patient that he never dreamt. I wondered that maybe he did not want to be in touch with such parts of his mind. He then revealed that he really felt that his life was just some sort of front and that he needed to put on a kind of "salesman act" to cover things up. He said that he would run his fingers through his hair and stroke his chin in order to try to prevent people looking at his spasms of torticollis. Yet beneath this he felt himself to be an empty character. Mr G was so fearful of his violent phantasies that he lived in isolation in as objectless a world as he could make. He described his life as empty, and he was devoid of friends. He was revolted if people brushed against him. When I commented on how I had not felt such a reaction from him when we had been talking together earlier, he told me that he regarded me as a non-person. I replied that it seemed to be safer for him to perceive me in a non-person position, and he replied, "Yes, that's the crux of it."

The patient's non-dream was a pointer to enormous repression and to the shutting out of any knowledge, leaving a blank space. His torticollis was mirrored by an internal twisting of his mind that he defended against by "blanking off". In the place of a dream, and for the first time in the consultation, this gap revealed his "front", and this metaphor could then be examined—or, more realistically, avoided by him. This man was severely ill. He had spasmodic torticollis and was paranoid of the world as a means of defending himself from having to have any contact with it. He had arrived quite late for the consultation and, hoping that he would miss his appointment, was indicating how fearful he was of getting in touch with himself, for fear of his own violence getting out of control. If I had begun by asking him questions, his central fear of violence may not have been uncovered in such a direct way. In fact, he gave many indications during the consultation that he should not be dynamically explored out of concern that he would become more overtly paranoid. Therapy outside of an inpatient psychiatric hospital would make it very hard to contain any potential regression towards more overt illness, especially in the gaps between the sessions. Here, the non-dream provided the greatest point of connection in the consultation. Whilst the patient was not suitable for dynamic treatment at that time, perhaps he left knowing that he had been able to communicate with an absence, allowing some understanding of his present difficulties. His fear of revealing any history indicated the possibility of massive early trauma in his life, such that he felt unsafe in the presence of others. He protected himself by living as a loner. The work we did together on the absent dream was a little more evocative for him than his defence against answering questions about his past.

Ms. H: aged 26—a dream dreamt just prior to the consultation

Following an overdose of fifty paracetamol, a psychiatrist referred the patient for an assessment for psychodynamic treatment. A young female journalist, Ms H, described feeling alienated, and that she had difficulty in asking for help, always expecting betrayal. She felt "out of control, eaten up, poisoned by her own bitterness". Ms H said that she had "grown up with a terrible mother" who she thought was probably both psychotic and alcoholic. Nonetheless, she herself seemed to have an active and quite successful career. She described having many anxiety dreams where, despite finding herself homeless, being a journalist meant that she still had to find news items for publication in the newspaper. In one dream some items had got lost and the copy could not be printed. I said that she appeared competent and got things done, but that beneath this surface she was describing a chaotic situation of things being lost, and of having no safe place. Following my interpretation, she remembered a specific dream from the previous weekend in which she was going on an outing for the newspaper and felt she would be murdered. I linked this association with her recent attack on herself with a near-fatal overdose, which had brought her to hospital and to the attention of the psychiatrist. She described that she was now feeling very afraid that she would kill off an inner, important part of herself and would have to continue living on as a shell of a coping person, dead to her feelings and to life. In speaking about this, she was also hoping to inform both of us that, rather than kill herself, she was expecting to survive her self-assault. Perhaps her fear of becoming a lifeless shell was actually how she unconsciously thought about her life prior to the overdose, rather than being the corresponding reaction to it later.

Her pull towards deadliness was apparent from her dream, as well as being repeated as a dream enactment in trying to murder herself. This provided evidence that important themes ran true in the dream she brought to the consultation, as she was very preoccupied with and fearful of her capacity for destructive rage. The dream also revealed, if one needed to see it more clearly, the still overt suicidal feelings of this young woman. Although that did not contraindicate therapy in itself, it was important to know that her capacity for self-harm was unabated, and was continuing in her subsequent dream life. There was also a transference aspect to note in the dream, going on an outing and fearful that she would be murdered. Attending the consultation would mean bringing her news stories, as associations, to the meeting that she was going to have with me. The idea of her being murdered can be thought of as having several meanings in addition to exposing her continuing suicidal tendency. A state of being murdered in the consultation might mean not being able to discuss the internal contents and stories in her mind—the killing of her desire to communicate. She was also unconsciously concerned that the interviewer would show no understanding and would murder her quest to find a safe place for herself.

Here we see the importance of the dream as a fulcrum that can allow a deeper exploration of the present state of destructive feelings. Clearly, an in-depth discussion of her feelings of destructiveness was a core component in assessing a suicidal patient for treatment. It was important to ascertain as much as possible the area of the patient that was utilising an act of self-harm, which had been survived, as a reason to undergo treatment, rather than to just re-enact the attempt on her life. The rest of the consultation focused on linking the outburst of actual aggression with the patient's early life experience and unconscious object-relational world. The value of her dream was its centrality to a theme of psychic murder, both now and as a representation of early childhood trauma, which could be further examined during the rest of the consultation.

Mr I: aged 30—a recurrent dream

A thirty-year-old man was described by the referring psychiatrist as vague, ruminating, unhappy, and isolated. His father had died when he was eight. This had the effect of apparently allowing him to feel free of paternal authority. Following his father's death, the family split up. He then stayed with his uncle's family for several years, whilst his siblings stayed with his mother. This was described as if a boy of eight years decides such matters, not wanting to admit that he was excluded from the rest of his family. When his father died, he essentially lost both of his parents and his siblings, this perhaps being the start of his state of isolation.

He described having lots of dreams, but could not remember any. I said that this absence implied that he was out of touch with that part of his mind. He said he had many recurrent dreams, but he could not remember the most recent. However, with difficulty and much thought, he was able to eventually tell me a recurrent dream. In the dream he was running along a path and scraped his left knee. He thought he might have done this by jumping over a boulder. It was the inside part of his knee that he had scrapped. He then said it was strange because he had recently been skiing and that was just the particular area that he had fallen on and hurt in reality. He said, rather vaguely, "Yes, I suppose that's how I do feel." He then remembered that when he first met his girlfriend, he cried because he somehow knew that nothing could come of it. "She had everything—parents, the right school, a decent life," very different from his life, which he regarded as a mess. He then said that I must not think that he blamed his father for dying, because that would be the easy way out. I said that he must feel very angry with his father who had not been around for most of his life, and he quietly agreed.

When pressed for a dream the patient was able to remember one, a dream in which he fell, was hurt, and wondered whether something was broken. I thought that the injury he sustained to his knee by jumping enabled the enactment of a manic façade of bravado that he had adopted in his life, in the dream covering up the scrape to his leg that somatically contained the sadness, distress, and rage caused by the breakup of the family when he was a child. This childhood event was the moment of his fall, the dream enabling a central emotional pivot of trauma to be revealed. Previously unable to remember anything, the patient was able to describe a particular dream which he had to acknowledge was deeply resonant with how he felt about his life, and with his anxiety about how broken he might still be after the early death of his father. He was even able to voice concern about feeling that nothing could come of a new relationship. He had expectations that any relationship that was meaningful to him would only be extinguished again. Such a revelation from his dream became valuable to him as a suggestion that subsequent therapeutic work might help him. Such a discovery would balance his internal nihilism of expecting nothing from life, and nothing from therapy. A patient with pessimism does not mean that dynamic treatment is contraindicated. Rather, it can be helpful for a patient to know and realise their negativity from the start, as a way of first forming a conviction of having a different and perhaps better life.

Mr J: aged 19—suicidal ideation and dream life

A man in his late adolescence was referred in some distress. He thought compulsively about problems and had been having episodes of anxiety for the previous two years. He also suffered from erectile dysfunction. Mr J had left the country where he lived and travelled around for a year before arriving in England. He quickly felt that he had collapsed and lost control of himself, although he remained, outwardly, seemingly well. Inside, he felt alienated from the world and was becoming more self-absorbed. He described suffering much deprivation as a child. He felt he hardly knew his father following the separation of his parents when he was seven. Prior to this the family had always moved around the world following his father's work, a pattern he had been unconsciously following on his recent meanderings. As a child he had lost a toe in a boating accident, and it had been sewn on again. His bland description of it as having been "nothing terrible" transmitted a horror. He was describing losing an important part of himself, and its impact, as it were, on his body. His present symptom of losing his erection was embodied in this metaphor that losing a toe was nothing. No erection was another no-thing.

He remembered a recurrent dream that took place in a very wide street where his mother lived. Three unknown men were in a car, and he joined them. The car accelerated faster and faster so that it was speeding at over a hundred miles an hour, and they were going to crash into a wall. A crash then did occur, and he was very surprised when he found that his death was really very pleasant, like a balloon slowly deflating. After a while I interpreted that perhaps the dream revealed the continuing nature of his life being out of control, and with frequent crashes, whilst he presented the outward appearance that it was a sort of enjoyable experience. He readily agreed to this, saying that he had never thought about it consciously. He talked about how he thought he was a vegetable. I said that it seemed he was describing how part of himself had died or was dead, in a vegetative state, and that his sense of retreating inside of himself was an attempt to protect himself, like the balloon, from awaking to painful things in his life. He accepted this interpretation, adding that he felt a strange pleasure in dreams of dying.

The important theme of suicide had, as yet, not entered the consultation, but in the dream it seemed very apparent, and there was quite a frightening pull towards destruction. In the crashing of the car into a wall, the dream is the vehicle to enable his aggression to be brought into the discourse. This has a considerably different resonance than the psychiatrist asking a surface question: "Are you still feeling suicidal?" Instead of feeling the terror and horror, the car crash was turned into something "pleasant, like a balloon slowly deflating". The example of his passive masochism was a valuable thing for him to experience and to notice. In the dream it is not he who is crashing, but rather the three men whose car he got into. He was not taking responsibility for his own destructiveness, but rather projecting it onto the others. The real accident with his toe was something that, alongside the dream, looked rather similar in structure, having all or part of his body castrated and then reattached not seeming to matter. The immediacy and horror of this dream was to be experienced by the listener, and perhaps indicated a borderline personality. This is an example of a splitting of the ego in which an individual defensively performs their bland affect by projecting their pain onto the listener. The patient went on to describe obsessional and paranoid thoughts, and was preoccupied with incestuous sexual phantasies. His dream in the consultation enabled a core sense of masochism to be revealed, an essential component to consider with his therapist in any subsequent treatment.

Mrs K: aged 23—a transference dream 1

Mrs K's parents were Jehovah's Witnesses and her referring doctor communicated that she had had a traumatic upbringing which she felt unable to discuss. What was salient in her questionnaire was her writing that her parents believed the end of the world was nigh, so there was no point in their children obtaining a proper education. The parents would tell potential converts how marvellous their religion and faith was, but on returning home they would both be very physically and emotionally violent to their child. The patient had described how she had been brought up to believe that the world was about to collapse, hearing the parental incantation that repentance was constantly required.

I met a pretty, diminutive, but very sad woman who, despite being forty, looked to be in her late teens. She had a lot of difficulty in starting to speak and found herself feeling intensely sad very quickly. She tried to cover this up with a cynicism that led her to comment dismissively on the box of tissues in the room. She could not make sense of her tears and said that people connected things with the past, but there was nothing to be done as the past was fixed—and anyway, her particular state was due to genetics. She added that she was terrified of becoming like her father, who was very depressed and had been hospitalised on several occasions because of manic-depressive illness. He had been given ECT in hospital. He was an impulsive man who was verbally aggressive. Her parents often argued, especially about money, and she remembered lying in bed as a child, listening to their rows and fearing that they would set the house on fire. She then went through a great denial that the past had anything to do with her sadness. She just had to make herself strong. I pointed out that it was she who had connected tears with her past. At once her resistance kicked in and she told me that that was what she had been expecting me to say. She did not think that talking could help at all. I replied that she had to decide if there was any point in giving me words for me to try to make sense of how she perceived her confused state.

Despite being cynical about my request for a dream she was able to recall a recent one. She had dreamt about her first boyfriend from when she was sixteen, meeting him at the top of a huge white building. She thought that the scene might have taken place in Italy where it was sunny. She had been desperate for the man to take notice of her but was unsure whether he would. Her associations were that it had been essential to be recognised by this boy who had been her first crush. I wondered if that first boyfriend had been a way for her to imagine being rescued from her family. She then said, "That would be a terrible basis for any sort of relationship, wouldn't it?" At the time I was in a large building, and one which was painted white. She seemed to be inviting me with the dream to be in a sunny place with her, perhaps also wishing for a rescue from her internal darkness, "desperate for a man to notice her". Despite her cynicism I felt that she was describing a great anxiety that I should notice her and her predicaments. Her comment that possible rescue was a terrible basis for a relationship could now be considered further. Did the idea of help mean that she should come and be seen but remain cynical about the process of the consultation? That would indeed have been a realistic expectation, following her description of her parent's model—outside of home a religious goodwill, but a darker side on returning home. Perhaps this had formed her cynicism, the impact of her parents being projected onto the consultation, the expectation being that worse would follow when she returned home. There was a good atmosphere in the dream, high up on the building, but this would later require a descent to the street. The dream structure contained the essence of a moment of transference in which she expected the consultation to be a repetition of her proselytising parents—something that would definitely not help, and that would perhaps be a repetition of her upbringing, by bringing her down.

She had an ambivalent hope but had lived a life in which she always returned to a traumatised self. The dream had evoked a core conflict that linked with her expectation that nothing which followed would be witnessed—and especially with her deeply entrenched cynicism that nothing could help in the future. Here, she was unconsciously projecting a future nihilism instead of realising that tragedy had already happened to her, and, with this fixed structure, there was a sense that nothing more could be developed during the rest of the consultation.

Treatment would be worthwhile if she dared to hope that it would deal with her dark expectations of the future. The evocative dream allowed many links to be available for the description of her negative state of mind. It made manifest her fear of being with people like her parents who spoke inauthentically about hope. Yet the dream opened up possibilities in the consultation, gradually allowing the depth of her nihilism to be observed and discussed.

Miss L: aged 25—a transference dream 2

A young woman was referred because she was obsessed with her spotty face, despite there being no marks or blemishes that could be seen by the observer. She readily presented a dream from the previous night about attending her consultation the following day! She dreamt that when she entered my room there were a dozen medical students, each with a copy of her questionnaire. She collected them all up and then left. This dream showed the immediate and transient transference that was established, dreaming of me prior to seeing me, although she did not appear to notice the discrepancy between her dream life and her actual experience of being in the consultation. At once there was a blurring of phantasy and reality as the dream revealed that her phantasy of seeing me and the reality of being there were in no way different. If there had been differences she might have commented that I looked different in the dream to how I was in reality. To my mind this pointed to a psychotic process, it seeming to her that I appeared just as she had dreamt me. In addition, the need to immediately collect back the questionnaires in the dream indicated paranoia. I interpreted that it was very difficult for her to show any knowledge about herself or her feelings, wanting straight away to take back all of the information. She agreed at once and added that she was afraid I would tell her to "snap out of it". In this context I felt that her use of the word "snap" was also indicative of her fragility and her potential to fragment into pieces. Her presenting symptom of having badly pocked facial skin—which she thought everyone could see, and of which she was ashamed—seemed to be a somatisation, despite nothing being visible, of her being mentally scarred. The dream enabled an understanding of this patient's great fragility, it seeming that her facial symptoms were holding her together, and away from a severe breakdown. This allowed us to work, in the remainder of the consultation, on how ill she felt herself to be beneath her skin.

Mrs M: aged 40—a transference dream 3

A forty-year-old woman came for a consultation with much anxiety about her daughter, who had recently tried to commit suicide. She explained that neither her own deprived and miserable childhood, nor bringing up her daughter for many years in a same-sex household, had any connection at all with the latter's present difficulties (a rather good example of negation). She had just dreamt about a very dear friend of hers who had recently (in real life) received a diagnosis of cancer of the tongue. Despite having half of her tongue resected there had been a cancerous spread to the larynx. The friend was unable to talk, but in the patient's dream they had been speaking on the phone. The patient added that she herself was slightly deaf. She seemed to perhaps have a slight difficulty in hearing me as well. And so the dream consisted of her talking with her friend, who could not speak, whilst at the same time being unable to hear her anyway. There was then a dream resolution without speech and hearing in which both of them looked into a mirror. In this way, the patient found that she and her friend could speak to each other and, in addition, that at the end of the conversation she was able to touch her friend, to her surprise feeling her through the mirror. In the dream she said, "Well, if I go through the mirror, I could be with you."

She then said that she had told this dream to colleagues at work but that nobody seemed to be interested. "That is how it is at work", she said. She would go in and say that her daughter had tried to commit suicide and everyone would carry on with their work. I wondered if she was perhaps also describing her own distance from her daughter's state of mind, and she agreed. The dream could be seen to have been an eloquent statement of the difficulty of making contact with someone who could not speak or hear—actually a statement about herself. She desperately wanted to communicate and to go against the flow of a defensive system, which she had earlier described as being like steel doors around herself.

In the dream she tried to communicate by looking into a mirror. I interpreted that by so doing she would only get a reflection of herself. This seemed to be a reflection of a constant self-assurance that perhaps she felt she had received from her mother when she was a baby, as well as being what she seemed to give her daughter, and what she expected from me. In other words, what became visible in the mirror of the dream were her narcissistic defences. The importance of her being able to tell this dream to someone and have some sense made of it, in contrast to the expectation of the people at work who ignored it, was that she was then, for the first time, able to take the consultation seriously. Now she was able to start looking at her own damaged childhood, which until that point in the consultation had been dismissed, unspoken, and unheard. This was a bridge to starting to make sense of her daughter's recent suicide attempt, towards which, despite her apparent concern, she was shown be emotionally shut off. In the dream the cancer that her friend suffered also stood for her daughter's near death. Up to this point the patient had been very removed from the connections and affect of her story. Investigating her dream allowed emotional connections that could enable work to begin in the consultation.

This case is a good example of how it is possible that a dream, despite its complexity, can be of clinical use. The patient might be reached psychically in the moment, rather than the assessor just listening passively to a litany of concern brought by a highly defended patient, lacking the emotional tools to comprehend their anxieties. As one becomes more competent at managing the complexities of the consultation by utilising one's own free associations, the material can be scanned for connections between the past and the present, and for affect. Very often one of these vertices are damaged—or sometimes both are, as in this case—emotional insight guarded against by a robust defensive organisation. Yet the free play of listening enables the assessor to realise the pivotal moment at which the patient starts noticing their attempts to prevent something they feel to be dangerous from appearing from beneath the surface. If the emergence of such moments can be enabled, the patient, whilst still maintaining their defences, can start to sense other states, such as sadness, and experience a real understanding of the authenticity of such events as they are discovered inside of themselves—not just following some direction set by the outsider. Such crucial moments can emerge in the first few minutes, when, for instance, a patient suddenly and unexpectedly bursts into tears—at the relief that there is an available other to listen. Or they can be found in the evocations of the early memory. A dream is also a good place to find unconscious emotional connectivity, although if this has to wait for the dream it can be a reflection of the distance of a patient from their unconscious life, due to the proliferation of defence. Even so, finding the beginnings of a deeper understanding in an incomprehensible dream, which colleagues at work had ignored (meaning they had ignored her), can be a profound moment in the life of someone who thinks that no one could ever understand them—an important relic of childhood containing a core truth about traumatic early years.

* * *

These specific fragments of dream life taken from the long interview are designed to show the value of looking together at dream formation. Each of the examples reveals the effectiveness of the dream structure in delineating areas of difficulty in relationships, early life, problems of affect, and their defensive structures. The dream in the consultation can open up the field, develop curiosity, and produce more of the patient's history from out of its threads. The dream also gives the patient a sense that their unconscious life is interesting, that it bears on their conscious difficulties in life, and that with time it can be understood. Moreover, it can link a symptom that appears to stand in isolation in their life to a whole system of unconscious object relationships, as well as repressed affects. The task is not particularly to do dream-analytic work per se, but rather to use the dream in the consultation as a particular form of thinking that links the patient's sleep life, history, early object relations, and affect system in a way that can be inclusive and helpful. It is especially useful when placed next to the early memory. Here, the developing hypotheses in the mind of the assessor can be tested. If the clinical material in each strand seems to be arranged in a similar direction, or if the early memory further informs the dream, or the development of each enables further pieces of remembered history to emerge, then the patient can begin to feel the pathways of a free-associative network as having some authenticity. Often the patient responds with the desire for further dynamic help, leading to a discussion of different forms of treatment. Even in those patients with great disdain for or resistance towards analytic thought, realisation can subsequently grow, even long after the interview, that there is a problem in their own mind, even if other, perhaps external factors are still blamed. A pre-existing determination to minimise the effect of such a meeting can still sometimes be joined by an idea that another person might, perhaps, understand them.

CHAPTER TEN

The sexual life of the patient

It is a most unfortunate thing that clinical medicine ignores one of the most pathogenic factors or at least hints at it delicately. This is certainly a subject in which the acquired knowledge of experienced physicians should be communicated to their juniors, who as a rule blindly overlook sexuality—at all events as far as their patients are concerned.

—Josef Breuer, in *Studies on Hysteria* (Freud & Breuer, 1895d,
p. 246 n. 1)

It is important for the assessor to develop the clinical skills that allow them to bear investigating the sexual life of patients. This is often a fruitful arena of exploration and can enable the assessor to get a grasp on how the patient unconsciously uses—or would wish to use—sexual relationships with the other. Sexual phantasy adds depth and meaningfulness to the understanding of an individual's character. In psychiatry, the diagnosis of personality disorder is often applied without ascertaining that much about the actual personhood of the patient. To the dream and the memories of early life a third polarity can now be added: the sexual life of the patient, in both phantasy and reality. To my mind it is the coming together of these three strands in the process of the assessment, and the entwining of their differing perspectives, that we might call the character of the person. The delineation of the individual system of unconscious object relationships begins here—in particular of the psychosexual dynamic, including both the specifics of conscious desire along with the unconscious sexual states of phantasy.

The sexual life in reality and also in the masturbatory phantasy is a specific gauge of the analytic percept "who is doing what, to whom, and why". A person's object-relationship system, as found in the early memory and in the dream, includes sets of relations populated by various internal characters, interacting and affecting each other in particular ways. Sexual desire is often a very delicate area of private life, and requires sensitive handling. Often it is not necessary to examine this part of the patient's mind in the consultation, especially if the clinical understanding developed so far has become increasingly clearer moving through the start of the consultation, the early memory, and the dream. It may well be that one has gained enough confidence from such areas that it is unlikely that re-examining psychic life through the prism of sexuality will add much more to the clinical impression at that time. Instead, sexuality as a specific topic can be left to find its place later in the unfolding of an analytic treatment. Sometimes, the patient aware of a dissonance in their sexual life will be brave enough to speak his or her concerns. For others it is too private and intimate a part of the mind to bear revealing so quickly during a consultation. The clinical temperature therefore needs to be taken in relation to the investigation of sexual life. Nonetheless, cultural awareness of the importance that psychoanalysis places on sexuality means that the patient usually expects the subject to be discussed. This is so ubiquitous that patients often also expect their psychiatrist to be interested in the sexuality in their life. It is useful for the subject of sexuality to be approached in an ordinary clinical way, similar to the professional way that a physician examines the body of their patient, including, when appropriate, the genitals. One is assisted, in the same way that the physician usually is, by the patient's expectations of the assessment. In fact, the patient may well feel that a vital part of themselves has not had a hearing if their sexual life is inappropriately left out of the consultation. This could also lead to thoughts about whether the assessor is able to face the patient's sexual mind or not, and to anxiety about whether the patient will really be understood.

Of course a particular strain in this area is in the development of the assessor's own sexual life. If we digress for a moment to junior colleagues learning to do consultation work, their personal world is, of course, private. However, if such privacy hinders the doctor's capacity to develop an appropriate doctor–patient relationship, then it becomes a delicately difficult area of their training. An obvious example would be a particular trainee's anxieties about the homosexual patient, possibly speaking more about their own sexual anxieties, projected onto the other, than the patient's (a good example of the impact on a doctor of a patient's unconsciously enacted sexuality, increased by the recipient's own sexual muddle, is to be found in Case 8 in the earlier chapter on Balint groups (pp. 87–90). More insidious is the disgust that a therapist or analyst can have in relation to their patient's clinical material, a reaction that might get in the way of their capacity for concern.

The discussion of sexual life is also an area where one can assess potential dangerousness and perversion in the patient. I shall give a brief example of a seemingly ordinary but depressed man who was able to describe in the consultation his sexual phantasy of tying a woman up and raping her to the point of his orgasm. At this moment of describing his exciting phantasy he imagined putting his hands around her neck as he tightened his grip. In the telling of his aggressive phantasy in the consultation he actually squeezed his hands together, causing me to feel a chill in my countertransference at that moment. His somatisation of strangling his object of desire had been brought into the consultation in a living and sadistic form. This was an indication that I needed to be alarmed at the prospect of his behaviour having a capacity to be enacted, having already entered the realm of bodily enactment in the assessment, rather than being kept in the mind. His excitement had developed into an action as he performed his desire in front of me. The discussion could be made use of, however, as the patient could be appropriately invited to examine his own anxieties about his sense of murderousness, as well as his despair at his feared lack of control. This led to a frank discussion about the sort of specialist treatment required—in this case a referral to the Portman Clinic in London, which specialises in perversion and criminality. Here it is important to give careful thought to such a specialist referral, rather than just referring to "the next therapist with a vacancy". The patient can then be directed towards real concern for their care and safety, preventing the possibility of them hiding the problem area, and preventing something far more frightening happening if the patient finds the assessment process leaving them vulnerable and unheld. If the patient currently being discussed wanted to explore his violence and misogyny, then it would be necessary that the therapist would not be in a position of feeling overwhelming anxiety. In a practical sense a male therapist would be more sensible, as well as the requirement of treatment taking place in a clinic or centre rather than an isolated private practice. These are important practical considerations following the emergence of violent sexual material. It does not necessarily mean that such a patient is untreatable if the boundaries and the therapeutic holding environment are well thought out in advance. This is a very strong reason for ascertaining the sexual life of some patients in the consultation.

Sexual phantasy is ubiquitous. A person who denies the capacity for such mental phenomena is not in touch with truth, revealing a great resistance to a part of their mental functioning. This can mean being out of touch with the other in the world. In investigating the masturbatory phantasy, it is interesting to hear whether it involves only the self or whether it involves another person or a part-object, such as a shoe or a glove (the excitement of involvement with a thing rather than a person), which plays its important part in fetishistic performance. One can begin to evaluate the importance of an oedipal dynamic, or whether the sexual phantasy is more a holding-on to a part or thing, the degree of which indicates how much it is derived from earlier one- or two-person psychology. In one-person psychological states of mind, the mental representation of the other may not exist. Here, the fetishistic part-object is of much more interest and importance than the presence of another person. This is very important later in the elucidation of the transference–countertransference, if treatment is thought to be a viable option.

Some writers have stressed the importance of discovering a specific underlying theme of sexual phantasy (Laufer, 1976). What I think is more important in the moment, however, is the specificity of a particular phantasy and its use in the assessment dialogue. What one person is doing to or with another in the drama of such phantasies is a disguise for the particular variations of the feelings of love and hate in the early relationships of the patient (Freud, 1919e). In 1933, in Ferenczi's influential paper on the "Confusion of Tongues between the Adult and the Child", we find the opening out of the field of perverse sexuality in his understanding that actual sexual trauma and physical and mental assaults on the child can have a great psychic impact in early life, as well as on the development of character. A much more detailed account of the underlying theory of early trauma can be found in my book *Landscapes of the Dark* (2011), where descriptions of the sexual violence and perverse mentation found in some patients are found to be rooted in profound early traumas, involving being hated and being the recipient of violence. Finding indications of such difficult sexual states of mind in an assessment can be the start of a profound understanding, then, and one that, if analysis is pursued, can be transformative. It is helpful for the therapist to have some skeletal idea in advance of the clinical sexual/ violent terrain that might need exploration, rather than unexpectedly happening upon perverse and even violent material later in treatment. Whilst stumbling over such difficult material is not uncommon in treatment, finding its early resonance in the assessment can only be helpful.

To complicate the argument, perversion functions in a similar and parallel state to Winnicott's transitional object (1951), but in the negative register. For Khan, "perversion-formations are much nearer to cultural artefacts than disease syndromes as such" (1979, p. 121). He goes on to describe the individual's life in a sort of total system that is very different from the clinical pictures seen in the neuroses and psychoses of many patients with psychiatric illness. This means that perverse formations are often much more difficult to perceive in the lives of some patients as the phenomena can be very split off, performed in "another life", as it were, and thus concealed. It is more likely that frank, enacted perverse life is not easily revealed in the consultation, but can sometimes be glimpsed in material in which someone is a watcher on some enacted scene. An example would be in a clinical account of Khan's (ibid., pp. 122–133): a patient too anxious to travel alone brought her au pair to the consultation, who was then required to sit in on the assessment! Khan accepted without questioning or disturbing its happening, allowing the potential revelations of a particular behaviour being brought to the meeting. During the assessment, it was the au pair who became dejected, apathetic, and anxious, whilst her mistress spoke with surprising ease about her own life. Khan could not examine much of the patient's personal life with a third person listening in the room. However, letting the patient bring herself to the assessment in that specific way not only allowed the patient to start an analysis without being too frightened but rather, by noticing the urgency of the split affect between the two, Khan was able to begin the analytic work with some sense that perverse functioning was at the origin of the dysfunction. The enacted splitting mechanism revealed a hidden state of the patient, with a historical mother and daughter and a projective-introjective system that was strict and complex. This case highlights the great value that performance of early object relations can have, specifically in relation to assisting evaluation of a potential perversion structure, as a secretly offered lead.

I now want to discuss some clinical material that on the surface looks like a perversion. It is less concerned with sadism and hate, however, than with a sudden narrowing of object-choice that, when eventually revealed and understood, allowed considerable change to develop.

A clinical vignette of the sexual life of the patient

Mr N: aged 64—a concealed sexual problem

This old, local farmer had been an inpatient on the professor's psychiatric unit for a year, with an unremitting and severe depression. Before being admitted he had taken a very large overdose of a mixture of antidepressants and painkillers. Finding himself alive following the overdose, he had tried to hang himself in one of the barns on his farm a few days later, but was found by a farmhand. These severe actions precipitated his admission to the psychiatric unit. Here, he had been given all manner of antidepressant medication, in many combinations and in increasing strength, as well as ECT, but to no avail. Despite an expectation that an analytic consultation would prove similarly ineffective, the patient had now been referred for such a consultation.

Mr N looked anxious and despairing. His general appearance, despite (or as well as) being an inpatient, was dishevelled, and he looked considerably older than his age of sixty-four years. His father had also been a farmer, and he had grown up on the farm that he had later inherited. He spoke about his past life and present hopelessness with a flat affect and with a degree of boredom. He gave no sense as to why he had taken the overdose and could give no account of the overwhelming depression, which had seemingly just struck him out of the blue. He had no earlier history of suicidal behaviour and this was his first breakdown. He had clearly been very suicidal at admission, and this had not altered a year on. One salient feature was his lack of will to engage in the process of the consultation, which he had been sent to have. It was the psychiatric team that were nonplussed that after a year of inpatient treatment the patient was in the same position. The professor had demanded a psychotherapeutic consultation, and the patient attended passively. Mr N had a total lack of any curiosity about his predicament, and instead had an aura of acceptance of it. Indeed, he was so disengaged as to resign from any active participation in his own life, preferring to continue in a state of regression by being cared for by the psychiatric nurses—in his view, forever. Returning to his farm was of no interest to him. As he was giving no spontaneity to telling his story, or to telling of his early family life, the consultation was grinding towards a stuck state. In my countertransference, I experienced his mood as having no interest in cooperating, or in understanding his present state of mind. Rather, I felt he wanted me to tire of his depressive passivity and to return him back to the ward. It was fair to say that he was highly defended.

His referral to the psychotherapy department was, as already indicated, around the anniversary of his admission, and this led me to ask him what had been happening in his life just prior to his suicide attempts. After a long pause he said it had followed the death of his wife. She had been ill for some months prior to dying. He began crying. They had married young and she had been a wonderful companion for some forty years. They were very compatible with each other in every way, running the farm together, and as lovers. He felt lost without her and was clearly bereft. The direction the consultation was taking was one of an unresolved mourning. Despite the emergence of this clinical material, though, this did not make sense of his intense resistance to knowing more about his state of mind.

At this point I asked him how managing on his own had affected his sexual life. At once he turned red in the face and began to sob. After a few moments I invited him to talk to me about this. He began by telling me more about his wife being his perfect companion, but he then went further, recounting her demand close to her death that he should have no other women after her. Loving her so much, he readily promised. He began to moan. Gradually, and with much guilt and embarrassment, he recounted that a few weeks after her death he had found himself sleepwalking. To his sudden horror he had awoken in the middle of the night and found himself in the nearby barn where he kept his pigs. With enormous shame he told me that he thought that, as he awoke, he had been having sex with a sow. He was desperately upset but he had also become "animated" for the first time in our meeting. I said that it was a difficult promise for him to make that after his wife's death he should not consider loving or having a sexual life with another woman. He became thoughtful and added that he had always been a sexually active man, as well as always being faithful throughout the marriage. I said that the promise that she demanded might be considered to be very controlling, even a cruel injunction from the grave. He looked at me for the first time and asked if I really meant what I had just said. I replied that another way to think of love is that, following a wonderful marriage, the partner dying might consider that her husband deserved to continue having a living life, which could include having another loving relationship. Such a matter, far from attacking his dead wife, would be the continuation of his creative adventure—one that sadly his dying wife could not join him on.

It seemed that his only way to resolve the dilemma of the vow to not have sexual relations with another woman was to have sex with the animals on the farm. Despite this being an ego-alien matter for him, it is well known in farming circles that farmers do have sex with farm animals under particular circumstances from time to time. For him it was a way of dealing with his sexual arousal whilst staying faithful to his dead wife. At the end of the consultation he plaintively said, "So I can have another relationship?" I replied that, whilst his marriage had been, as he had said, wonderful, his wife had unfairly controlled his life after her death. He agreed that she had always been a controlling character, but said that this had suited him, as he did not feel himself to be very ambitious. He had not minded acquiescing over the many years to her views and her decisions about their life. Now he was beginning to have other thoughts about his future. He was now much more lively in the room than he had been for most of the consultation, and said he would think about our discussion a lot.

Hospitalisation had become a defensive device that organised several different difficulties for him. The sense of guilt for his perverse object-choice since his wife's death could be punished by incarceration in a psychiatric ward, and this kept him away from his anxiety that further episodes of sleepwalking might return him to the barn again. He was also looked after there, and this solved his concern that he would not be able to manage on his own. In fact, part of his desire to find a new partner was not only about sexual desire, but about having a woman who would care for him in daily life. More painful than anything, however, was his terrible distress and embarrassment about his nocturnal habit, which disgusted him. That he had been unwilling to talk about the serious reality of his predicament meant that he had not been able to mourn. The root of his severe depressive state lay here with pathological and unresolved mourning. Perhaps the invitation for a psychodynamic consultation by the professor of psychiatry came at a propitious time, around the first anniversary of Mr N's admission to the ward. The power of the anniversary reaction and its impetus for enabling reminiscences allowed a weakening of his resolve to be silent. More than anything, however, the context of being able to open up a discourse about his sexual life within the context of a psychodynamic consultation enabled free-associative material to emerge. For the previous year, no staff member had been interested enough in listening to him about his life, enabling him to sink further into the depressive state that protected him from a return to reality. His defences had deterred everyone from communicating with him further, which he welcomed as he sunk further into regression. Yet his very facing of the reality of his wife's death, her control, and her prohibition on any relationship with a different woman—leading to his perverse nightmare solution—was the way in which he could begin to consolidate his mind, and in which he could mourn and begin to organise a possible recovery.

This is an example of the usefulness of sometimes entering a discourse on the sexual in the life of the patient. In this instance, it opened up the clinical picture and led to a relatively easy resolution—once he had dared to speak to another person about his guilty secret. The patient returned two weeks later for a further appointment and was considerably improved, on the brink of leaving the hospital having had arrangements made for a housekeeper to be taken on at the farm. Arguably, it could be considered to have been a transference cure, as no further treatment was required. Progress was left to his finding new solutions to the future, beyond his wife's control. Perhaps he had been able to replace his wife's negative control with my more benign statement that another relationship would not be an attack on his first love. As for the professorial unit, despite the helpful discharge of one of their impossible chronic cases—which they had been unable to treat in spite of various medications over a very long stay as an inpatient—they showed little interest in learning about the complex dynamics. This was a sad example of a form of British psychiatry that finds psychoanalytic ideas to be irrelevant and useless in the clinical encounter, despite psychiatry and pharmacology being able to give no answers in this particular case. The idea that psychoanalytic thinking and its clinical atmosphere helped to bring out and understand the history of a psychiatric case was ignored. Perhaps the discovery that the scientific vision—which diagnosed a severe depression only amenable to pharmaceutical treatment, and which was utterly disconnected from listening to the patient's account—was based on phantasy created too much instability in the clinical dogma and psychiatric ethos of the unit.

This was not a case of perversion, although there was some perverse object-functioning. Mr N was in a severe depressive state due to his failure to mourn the death of his wife, as well as his guilt at fighting her injunction to, like her, have no further sexual life. Whilst further analysis would have examined his passive masochistic position in relation to his controlling wife, as a re-enactment of his early object relations, this was unnecessary, the consultation having provided him with enough psychic energy and hope that he could return to living his life. Sometimes a consultation can do just that.

CHAPTER ELEVEN

Thoughts on the ending

Strange old man
Shall I go with you?
Will you to my songs
Play the hurdy-gurdy?

—Wilhelm Müller, "*The Hurdy-Gurdy Man*" (1824, p. 463)

We need to consider and evaluate how the work of the assessment up to this point has evolved in each of its two participants, and how it has been understood and imagined. By this time, the patient is beginning to have a sense of participating in an analytical dialogue. And it is becoming apparent how the patient is entering the process: how they have started to think about their early family structures, their early memories, the development of ideas from their dream world, and perhaps the connection of their sexual life with the way that they experience their unconscious object world. How does the patient take to such explorations? Do such matters make a new sort of sense, or contain an atmosphere of unthought known? If so, is the work of thinking together syntonic, accepted as having an authenticity concerning the emergent description the self? If this is the case, the

193

patient may be in a quiet and thoughtful state and, using Balint's term, in an *arglos* state of receptivity. Whilst the patient will have an anxiety about their need to seek a consultation due to disturbances to their life, the exploratory atmosphere created in the consultation may contain some realisation of having been heard, and even understood somewhat. This in itself may be a new state, especially as many arrive in a state of feeling that they have always looked after themselves on their own. By this I mean that their life trajectory has developed out of early traumatic states in which the accumulation of slights and of being uncared for has led to the development of a one-person psychology, a "me against the world" position, expecting the other not to understand—because they never did.

Or the consultation may find that some symptom formation has been refracted through their early life, and that there are connections between neurotic and psychosomatic symptoms, again leading to some hope that their difficulties in life can be meaningful within the context of their life's history and relationships. The patient may begin to think that their symptoms can be thought about in new ways, in particular in cooperation with a therapist. They have thought as deeply as possible about their problems and symptomatic existence long before they decide to attend for a consultation. Yet thinking alone, to oneself, is far from speaking one's mind and dream to the other. The enormous importance of the move from solipsism to dialogic thought with the other, in a dyad, should not be underestimated. The patient's rehearsal of thoughts in the privacy of their mind is very different to speaking them to another, and to hearing themselves speak from outside of the self. Now it can be ascertained whether the patient can bear not only an awareness of discovery with the other, but also their revelations and thoughts being taken out of the privacy of the self. Such a privacy has a relative safety, perhaps, but can be a primary cause of the continuation of the neurosis—for instance, the farmer, who, by not speaking about the aftermath of his wife's death, maintained a ghostly existence within a psychiatric unit for over a year, this avoidance being psychically safer than divulging his humiliating solution to deal with his loss. Daring to breach the security of the self is certainly painful, but it can also bring relief, potential for psychic change, and the possibility of resuming a developmental process and a creative life, previously stalled by the stasis of an illness.

Meanwhile, the assessor begins to develop a psychodynamic hypothesis that links the presenting symptoms with the character of the patient within the context of their early life history. There is a sort of coherence between the different groups of phenomena in the early memory, the dream, and the affect system that has been developing in parallel to the way in which the transference and countertransference have emerged. At this stage it would be wrong for the assessor to assume to know the treatment desire for the patient, however. Now would be an appropriate time to enquire how the patient imagines continuing with the matters that they had been discussing together. There can be a return of a resistance to change here, as the idea of having treatment really emerges. The patient that makes clear at the start that their day is so full and busy that there is really no space for therapy needs to decide about the time and cost of incorporating a treatment process. A more meaningful way of understanding such a position is that, for such patients, every lacuna of life has to be filled in an attempt to prevent the return of the repressed. Following the work of the assessment, the patient may be aware of having a choice. There is no demand from the consultant that they undergo the rigour of a treatment. Knowing that there is a potential may suffice for some. Or a patient may feel that treatment is not appropriate now, but that it might be possible in the future. There is nothing wrong with such an outcome, leaving the patient to mull over where they have been in their experience of the consultation. They may need to think about this later.

For others, the receptivity of the process lends weight to the possibility of beginning to trust in the idea of exploring psychic life in a psychodynamic treatment setting. Work needs to be done to find out what they imagine of treatment, as well as what may be appropriate and possible. Most of us would prefer the simplest solution, perhaps once-weekly therapy for a few weeks. But, depending on the severity of the illness, its longevity, and perhaps its recalcitrance, more complex treatment may be necessary. The consultation may be seen as a *hors d'oeuvre*, a taster of the terrain (both historical and traumatic) that can be discovered in a freely associative way in the "talking cure". The more complex the diagnosis, the lengthier the cure—as in much of medicine. If the symptoms have certain roots in early life, then this implies that the material resonates through that person's life, but it also points to the complexity of such states of defence, perhaps in use for many decades.

This can mean that many more connections with events and phantasies, in that constellation of object relationships, need to be spun out and known. For instance, while the depressed farmer in his unresolved mourning was certainly able to make a move from his hospital life, he might be concerned in the future about having a new relationship that could reawaken a defensive acceptance of his dead wife's demand. Or he may want to think out the meanings of his passivity in relation to a woman, and how this might reflect his unconscious view of his parents' marriage, or a bringing into the present tense of a dominant mother, or an identification with a passive father, or similar enactments in relation to siblings. Such variables precipitate complexity, indicating the necessity for a longer and deeper treatment so that more can be understood and character change can be more effective.

It was Reich (1933) who began to direct attention beyond the symptoms of neurosis, anxiety, depression, obsessionality, paranoia, and a range of psychosomatic disorders, to the way that such psychic defences become bound up in the characters we grow into. Character analysis underpins much of modern-day psychoanalysis and requires the intensity of an analysis over several years in order to examine the complex web of events, history, imagination, phantasy life, *après coup*, and day and night dreams that are the constellations of our unconscious life. Such a radical journey often leads to the development of what Balint called a "new beginning" (see Balint, 1968, pp. 131–148). Some patients desire to engage in such a direction. If psychoanalysis is desired, some time needs to be given in the consultation to look at how it might be achieved. Can it be afforded? Might they be directed to a low-fee clinic at an institute of psychoanalysis? Can time be made within a busy life for daily sessions? Can they attend sessions before work, or after? Is flexitime at work a possibility? All such ideas are important to evaluate whilst simultaneously testing the strength of resistance to a therapeutic direction. A desire for analysis inevitably comes with a sense of the impossibility of letting such a commitment into one's life, and of sustaining it for the full length of its process; such is the inevitable paradox in the wish to undergo an analysis. At this point in the process it is very helpful to enquire what type of treatment has been imagined. This in itself can indicate much about a patient's passive position of wanting someone, the grown up, to take responsibility and to make it better. Speaking about this may help the patient to realise that they hold the responsibility for their life and its trajectory. While this may mean that they have a mountain to climb, albeit joined by a guide, it can also be an empowering position for them to take towards their future.

Sometimes the wish to have once-weekly treatment is firmly held. The assessor can then point to the various matters that have just been sketched out: the complexity of unconscious life meaning that only briefly engaging with such work will prevent the patient from fully exploring its depths. In addition, a great problem of once-weekly psychotherapy is that, by the time the patient has caught up with the week's happenings, there is often no time left in the session to go into further depth, into the complexities of thoughts and meanings, weekly treatment becoming a continual performance of catching up. Further, if a session is missed, then half a month will have gone by beyond the frame of treatment. If the patient can attend the next day, allowing the possibility of a dream between the sessions, there is a dynamic continuation from the previous day's session.

For some patient's the idea of the consultation leading to further treatment is a step too far. There is nothing wrong with having such a view, as it is important that the time is right to proceed with such a venture. Sometimes there is a certain amount of psychic gain if the patient is told that treatment is not recommended. It is invariably more honest and of greater value to add "at this present time", rather than to preclude such a treatment ever being possible. The patient may take comfort in being denied treatment, taking it to mean that they are too special, or that their defences are impenetrable. Others may be angry, despite being deeply resistant, that they are not offered treatment in order to continue a fight that may be very old in their life. In such cases I think there is wisdom in using the material from the assessment to demonstrate how they themselves have a deep reluctance to engage, rather than allowing them to project the negative onto the assessor. Mr C, who described the early memory of sand being thrown in the face, would be a pertinent example. Rather than just telling him that psychodynamic treatment was not suitable for him, my interpretation enabled him to grasp how difficult it was for him to receive help from another person without immediately defending his isolation by throwing sand. Leaving with some sense of responsibility for how he keeps the other at bay may enable him to consider this behaviour over time, and perhaps develop the bravery to attend again. It would also mean he would be less likely to use the assessment to increase his paranoia, as if the other person had stopped him from being treated. It is a false solution for the consultant to be seen to be the guardian of treatment, such that a patient may leave feeling aggrieved. The value in elucidating that the source of the "no" is within the patient, or, more accurately, that there is a character in their mind that is saying it—a rigid parent or a frightened child—is that this allows such causes to be thought about beyond the consultation. In time, such a person might re-apply in order to go further in attempting to overturn the "no", with its concomitant weight of deadness, and in daring to embrace a creative life—as Michael Parsons has recently commented (2014, p. 14), this is to overcome the problem of living a life that is not fully alive.

Whilst it is reasonable that some patients are unsuitable for psychodynamic treatment, it is important to ascertain if other treatments could be helpful. If anger management is a problem, in a character unable to examine their mental dynamics, it may be useful to ask the patient if they would be interested in a behavioural treatment involving a rule system, and not necessarily demanding a deep understanding of their life. Others may require psychiatric hospitalisation. It can happen that a medical practitioner, thinking that the patient is beyond their initial crisis, refers a patient that is actually still suicidal. During the assessment there may be much to indicate that the contemplation of suicide is still very active in the patient's mind. Then it is important to assess the level of danger and violence in the patient, as well as trying to understand the antecedent history of the suicidal thinking. The specific details of the suicide attempt are crucial. It is too perfunctory to accept a story that some tablets were taken, as this may just be a formula to conceal the amount of psychic violence still present. It is important to know how many tablets, and of what kind. And where was the attempt on their life made? There is a difference between taking an overdose alone in an isolated cottage and taking an overdose in one's bedroom while the rest of the family are at home. In such details, it is important to be able to distinguish instances in which the aggressive gesture may not be an expression of a deep desire to die, but rather a wish to disturb in order to be seen. Also, just because one is seeing a patient who has tried to commit suicide does not mean that they still want to. Clearly, it is also important to give thought in the consultation to the various possible meanings beyond the bland statement of a wish to die. More aggressive ways of attempting suicide indicate the level of the patient's violence. Is the patient a gun owner? Did they try to hang themselves? If so, was it connected with a particular form of masturbatory excitement that is felt by some men? Here the topic of violence and suicide brings us back to sex. When an amount of violence is ascertained in the clinical material, the rest of the assessment might still suggest that dynamic treatment could be valuable. In this case, my rule of thumb is that the more ill the patient the greater the need for intensive treatment, in order to psychically hold the patient. Waiting a whole week to see how the patient has managed in the gap, with the awareness of their disturbances, lays too much anxiety on the therapist, as well as leading the patient to perhaps wonder why they are not being treated more intensively, and to imagine that the therapist is not able to cope with them. Such is the twin danger of not considering the appropriate therapeutic arrangement in advance.

Curiously, in the realms of the unconscious it is far more likely that a patient will decide themselves the appropriate operation, in ways that would be inconceivable if they were having a consultation with a surgeon. It would be regarded as comic for such a patient to tell the specialist where to make an incision, and how long they will stay in hospital. Yet in the realm of mental life it is as if some patients must be the expert in the field of psychodynamics, even more knowledgeable than the specialist they consult. Such material can be discussed in order to elucidate whether this is another layer of anxiety or whether it suggests a pathological narcissism. Dynamically, such behaviour can reveal how the patient regards the other as inferior, and this may have much antecedent history, including that of the atmosphere of early object relationships.

It is important to consider the patient's ability to wait for a treatment vacancy, or if treatment needs to start quickly—even the following day, perhaps. If the patient is being assessed in a clinic, there is invariably a wait of weeks or months before a vacancy is available. If the patient can only make time in the early morning the availability will be further curtailed, as this time of day is in great demand. Arguably, a patient who is not employed might take any available time if it makes the start of treatment sooner. This is often a place for a resurgence of resistance and, if unexpected, this can undermine all that preceded, leading to a sudden impasse. The resistant state that has existed at various degrees through the consultation re-emerges in such moments near the end, often in relation to a frank discussion of the reality of therapy, and this is not an unexpected position. However, for an unemployed patient it is worth pausing to think about session times, as attending therapy during work hours may add to a resistance to work. This is perhaps something to give more consideration to further down the line, being less important than making a therapeutic start, but signalling it in advance has its value later on. One use of private analytic practice is that, if there is a suitable vacancy, it is possible to very quickly start work with the patient. Whilst most patients easily manage to wait a few weeks, to make time or to prepare for therapy to be part of their life, other patients will struggle. For instance, if they grew up in a perceived atmosphere in which nothing that grown-ups said was true, or if promises were never kept, then there is an urgent transference issue. In spite of the work of the consultation, a significant wait to begin treatment may harden the negative transference and be too much for the vulnerable patient to bear. Whilst such a structure invariably reoccurs throughout the treatment—at termly breaks, for example—taking such a mental expectation seriously at the beginning of treatment can very valuably underpin and strengthen the foundations for what follows.

By now it is clear how many diverse parameters need to be considered when setting the initial consultation, and perhaps it seems impossible to achieve all of this in one meeting. As a result of this time pressure, there is a long tradition of assessment being spread over more than one session, beginning with Freud, who sometimes found that it is useful for some patients to attend assessment interviews over a few weeks. Sometimes, however, within the frame of ninety minutes or two hours, and with an analyst practised in consultation, the full terrain can be covered. Sometimes it is worthwhile making a further appointment a week or so later, so that both assessor and patient can reflect on the process, and to see what the latter has made of the initial consultation: have more free-associative links been made, or has resistance blocked such paths?

Near the end of the consultation it is helpful to enquire what the patient has made of the experience, and whether it is what they had expected. It is also important that a small amount of time is left to enable the patient, in a state of *déshabillé*, to gather themselves together prior to departing. This is a time where the patient may speak of the unexpected nature of the dialogue and its effect on them. Some may be grateful for being helped to see beyond the horizons that they arrived with. Others may say it was all too predictable, indicating that they feel as competent as the analyst, as if engaged in a competition—perhaps another expression of their early history. Similarly, it is worth wondering how they will feel once they have left the consulting room, as they may reflect on being outside the thinking dyad and alone. Again, this picks up the motif of the patient being on their own again, here meaning that they have to take responsibility for remembering and thinking about what was discussed in the consultation. Difficulties at this point relate to the problem of being with another, and to the problem of being alone, and can have much traction if early issues of being alone predominated in their upbringing.

In concluding the assessment, the patient may have established what they require in terms of psychodynamic or other therapy, or they may want to consider their needs further—rather than to rush a decision, or to feel that they have to please the other (also reminiscent of earlier times). A further appointment can be made, or can be left for the patient to arrange at a later time.

Areas of resistance about taking up treatment

> No such thing
> as innocent
> bystanding.
>
> —Seamus Heaney, "Mycenae Lookout" (1996, p. 30)

If the patient desires and needs psychoanalytic or psychotherapeutic treatment, who are they referred to? In private practice, the decision is whether to take the patient into one's own practice. If so, then the difficult problem of the particular days and times of sessions will require consideration—as well as the cost. To begin with the scheduling, it may be unlikely that the analyst has many different times available. Even if the patient is in control of their work life, this does not mean they will wish to cede control to the other by accepting the analyst's timeframe. Nonetheless, with the offer of treatment comes the demand that the patient makes enough time available—for the fifty-minute hour, and to get to and from the appointment. For most people this is another part of the difficulty in deciding to accept treatment, yet it needs to be worked out. Often the sense of difficulty abuts the unconscious idea that things ought to be easy. Despite time being at a premium in modern life, however, it is possible to make space for analysis. If not, how can one return to the place where one has been living a less than satisfactory life, when now is the time to be brave and to take the imaginative leap—with some hope, following the depth interview—that one will be held and listened to?

If the consultant has no vacancy, then hopefully, having ascertained something of the internal world of the patient, a referral to a colleague of some sort of "good fit" will be possible. Often some disappointment is registered that treatment cannot be with the consultant. This disappointment may be real, especially if a good working relationship developed in the consultation, but the assessor needs to be aware that their narcissism is being stroked, treated as if they are the special therapist. The reality is that the patient needs us to do our best for them in arranging their future treatment. I usually say that I hope to refer them to a good analyst or therapist, but that, if they feel an instant impression that they cannot work with or tolerate that person, they can come back to me for another name. Such a sense is comparable to the primitive knowledge a baby has, through taste, that something is good enough to swallow, or whether it should be spat out. I do not offer the option of changing therapist weeks or months into the therapy, however, as any negativity will need to be worked out in the transference–countertransference of the ongoing work.

For patients with difficulty affording treatment, the possibility of being accepted for a reduced-fee scheme as part of the clinical activities of an analytic society can be very helpful. In this case, the patient cannot be referred to a particular therapist, but rather the "brick mother" (a term that plays on the holding suggested by the physical building) of an analytic institution, where the patient will need to undergo further assessment. I give this information to the patient, and also explain that treatment may require four or five sessions weekly for at least two years. The possibility of an intense and ongoing analytic treatment can then be afforded as the fee will be compatible with the patient's financial resources, subsidised by the clinic or by the trainee analyst who desires a training case. Someone not working and on social benefits may only need to pay £1 a session—a contribution, nonetheless. With the address and phone number of the institute, the patient can decide, in their own time, to make contact.

The particular fee for treatment is another hurdle. Some analysts make this an easy task for themselves by having a fixed and relatively low fee. This treats all patients in the same way, which is odd, especially as the assessment has accentuated their individuality. Such financial reasoning is based on a sort of socialist idea of not wanting to make money out of the neurotic. However, such pricing is often offered by senior analysts who bought their house decades ago, and whose grown-up children are no longer part of their monthly expenses. As one patient said to me, "I don't pay more for my loaf of bread than the next customer, even though I can afford more." One problem that can be indicated here is a core contempt for money, projected onto the therapist. Cut to the newly qualified analyst, however—with a mortgage and a young family, at the height of their need for money—and it is clear that there needs to be a better balance in valuing the work. Or, from the opposite perspective, if an analyst has a sliding scale for fees, why should the rich patient not be invited to pay a higher fee, knowing it can be easily afforded, or that such an increase is of no consequence? The rich patient is invariably on the lookout for being "ripped off", however. Work may need to be done to consider why they might prefer to pay a low fee for analysis while purchasing a new car every year and having expensive holidays. This usually suggests the low esteem in which they hold their mental products. It can helpful for this to be challenged, however, and for them to feel that they are in the hands of an experienced professional, rather than the cheapest. Their solicitor, surgeon, tailor, and architect would be expected to charge appropriately, and so should the therapist. Of course, both a fee too small and a fee too large could be perverse, and the therapist needs to be thoughtful about how they manage their practice. Taking a patient who can pay a good fee, however, can make it possible for another to have therapy at less cost. This is often a very difficult area to negotiate—some people can be even more inhibited to discuss money than to talk about sex! If one finds later in treatment that the agreed fee is too low or too high, it can be adjusted appropriately, in the same way that second thoughts can be valuable in more accurately establishing reality.

I have left until last the most important argument around money. Freud's theory of anal eroticism developed the idea of the potential for love to be projected onto faeces, which could then be stored up with constipation. This meant that the love, as faeces, was kept inside, resulting in a meanness of character. In relation to this it becomes apparent that ascertaining the fee may be part of the analytical task, rather than it being possible to just accept a particular fee in order to get on with the start of treatment. This is because money can be seen to be deeply connected to anality, ownership, and the line between mean and generous, as in withholding or letting go. These are analytic tasks to be discovered and understood, and the fee can sit intimately at the centre of them. Having a fixed fee leaves aside the unconscious meaning of wealth. I charged one of my first private patients a small fee as I felt that I was not particularly knowledgeable at the start of my training. The patient readily agreed to this. For several weeks, along with whatever else she communicated, she told me of the weekly cost of the hay for her stable of racehorses, unconsciously exposing her wealth. Eventually I enquired more of her life, and heard that as well as owning horses she had a Rolls Royce coupé that she parked a couple of streets away, as she thought that if I saw it I would overcharge her. Yet she had felt profound unconscious guilt about cheating me, motivating her hints about her wealth. Her guilt was easily analysed as it was attached on one level to discussing the fee, and resolved by raising the fee to a more appropriate amount. She did not have to pretend to be poor and yet she had come from an impoverished family, knew hardship, and had only met good fortune through the success of her husband's business. Her conflict, represented by money, was centred around her poor childhood and her negativity towards her husband—as, despite being financially generous to her, he was emotionally mean. The case suddenly opened up, no longer rigidly bound to the wrong fee.

CHAPTER TWELVE

Some conclusions

"It's no use going back to yesterday, because I was a different person then."

—Lewis Carroll, *Alice's Adventures in Wonderland* (1865, p. 109)

Whilst the model I have described is the underpinning of the work, it is not a blueprint that must be rigidly adhered to. It is a model that allows and calls for the complexity of examining several overlapping fields: the first moments of the consultation; the patient's account of their family life, an early memory, and a dream; and the end of the consultation. This clinical data is a blend of objective and subjective information, and a mixture of words, affects, and pictograms of scenes and situations. The assessment provides a rich multidimensional matrix in which the different spheres of discourse, as well as the patient's capacity to understand, develop trains of associations. The capacity to play with this stream of material casts a more living picture than a one-dimensional history-taking procedure, which leaves very little space for an encounter with the unconscious object relations and their concomitant anxieties.

One problem this book is therefore addressing in its return to Balint is that, for many reasons, therapists and analysts have received very little training in the subject of assessment. This is despite assessment being one of the key and most complex moments in the analytic process, especially as one needs to know, in the lightest way possible, about so many variables of mental life and history. It could almost be a subject for postgraduate study, as it requires knowledge of unconscious object relations, of states of affect, and of the intermingling of history and phantasy, as well as of the wide range of states of psychopathology. Neurotic illness, like depression, may derive from states of early loss of the object, developing into manic depression, or obsessional states with an interplay between mania and depression, alternating with the obsessions. It is beautifully described by Abraham (1924). The paper describes the patient unconsciously moving between defensive structures, moving from manic-depressive states to obsessional defences and back again, which initially appear to be in a tangled confusion. After further examination, however, these movements are shown to constitute a double-layered defensive system that needs to be viewed from both parameters of manic depression and obsessionality. In addition to neurosis, the psychopathologies of psychotic states need to be known, as do states of perversion. Psychosomatic states will also enter the diagnostic picture of many patients. From this perspective the field seems potentially overwhelming. How best to think about diagnostic frames, however provisional, in the face of the compelling and potentially infinite personal data waiting to be discovered in the course of analytic dialogue?

Perhaps the greatest impediment to this work is that most practitioners do not perform many assessments in a year, with too many colleagues possibly relying on more senior analysts to do the work of the assessment, being grateful that it has been done and the patient referred. In my observation, this does not obviate the receiving therapist from doing their own assessment. If there are important questions that emerge from the report then, at the start of the treatment perhaps, some matters can be explored further—or sometimes they can be left until later in the treatment, until they re-emerge. Either way, openness to the complexity of unconscious life starts from moment zero, like the silence out of which the first musical note appears—which for Daniel Barenboim is the first musical moment (personal communication, Seville, 2009)—before the analysis proper, as it might improperly be called, begins. I desire to give the last quotation to my colleague Michael Parsons:

Analytic listening has a special quality. It is not just a matter of carefully registering what a patient says, or waiting passively through a silence, for whatever they are going to say next. It is the active offering of a certain kind of attentiveness, which patients respond to just as much as they do to what the analyst says. It is by listening in this way, and seeing what happens in someone as a result of being listened to in this way, that an analyst senses what sort of capacity this person has to make use of analysis. The analyst's listening is also what gives patients, for their part, a sense of what psychoanalysis has to offer them, and of how important it feels to them to make it possible. What prospective patients respond to, I think, is a sense of being in contact with something they have not encountered before. They do not know what it is; they might find it hard to put into words; but the feeling of being attended to, with a kind of relaxed intensity at a very deep level, is absolutely distinct. In a consultation, what I would look for most of all is how someone responds to this sense of being in the presence of the other.

(Parsons, 2015, p. 21)

Like much in life, more experience of consultations leads to greater competency, as well as increased understanding of the many forms that psychopathology can take. At the heart of the complexity of consultation, however, is recognition of being in the presence of the other—for many the first time that they have been experienced by the other, and realised such a moment. To conclude, when Balint introduced psychoanalysis to medicine, he was asking doctors to take account of the unconscious aspects of their own practice. In so doing, he initiated a dialogue that goes profoundly against the grain of the forms of fact-checking, inflexible knowingness, and perceived medical control of the symptom, inscribed into medicine itself. Today, he can also be seen as issuing a warning to psychoanalysis, all the more relevant at a time when analysts are increasingly being asked to quantify their work. In the very first moments of clinical assessment, where analysis appears not yet to have begun, the temptation to limit the exchange to the world of facts and calculation is at its most tempting. Paradoxically, this is why assessment matters so much. The first dialogue either opens the way to the inner, most hidden recesses of the mind, or it does nothing.

REFERENCES

Abraham, K. (1924). Short study of the development of the libido, viewed in the light of mental disorders. In: D. Bryan & A. Strachey (Trans.), *Selected Papers of Karl Abraham, M.D.* (pp. 418–501). London: Hogarth, 1949.

American Psychiatric Association. (2013). *Diagnostic and Statistical Manual of Mental Disorders* (5th edn). Washington, DC: American Psychiatric Association.

Argelander, H. (1976). *The Initial Interview in Psychotherapy.* New York: Human Sciences.

Balint, A. (1939). Love for the mother and mother love. In: M. Balint, *Primary Love and Psycho-analytic Technique* (pp. 91–108). London: Tavistock, 1952 [reprinted 1965].

Balint, E. (1963a). On being empty of oneself. *International Journal of Psychoanalysis, 44*: 470–480.

Balint, E. (1963b). On being empty of oneself. In: J Mitchell & M. Parsons (Eds.), *Before I was I: Psychoanalysis and the Imagination* (pp. 37–55). London: Free Association, 1993.

Balint, E. (1968). The mirror and the receiver. In: J Mitchell & M. Parsons (Eds.), *Before I was I: Psychoanalysis and the Imagination* (pp. 57–62). London: Free Association, 1993.

Balint, E. (1987). Research, changes and development in Balint Groups. In: A. Elder & O. Samuel (Eds.), *While I'm Here, Doctor: A Study of the Doctor–Patient Relationship* (pp. 95–102). London: Tavistock.

Balint, E. (1989). Creative life. In: J. Mitchell & M. Parsons (Eds.), *Before I was I: Psychoanalysis and the Imagination* (pp. 99–108). London: Free Association, 1993.

Balint, E. (1993). Enid Balint interviewed by Juliet Mitchell. In: J Mitchell & M. Parsons (Eds.), *Before I was I: Psychoanalysis and the Imagination* (pp. 221–236). London: Free Association.

Balint, E., & Solomon, J. S. (Eds.). (1973). *Six Minutes for the Patient: Interactions in General Practice Consultation.* London: Tavistock.

Balint, M. (1947). On the psycho-analytic training system. In: *Primary Love and Psycho-analytic Technique* (pp. 257–262). London: Tavistock, 1952 [reprinted 1965].

Balint, M. (1950). Changing therapeutic aims and techniques in psychoanalysis. *International Journal of Psycho-analysis, 31*: 117–124.

Balint, M. (1952). New beginning and the paranoid and the depressive syndromes. In: *Primary Love and Psycho-analytic Technique* (pp. 230–252). London: Tavistock, 1952 [reprinted 1965].

Balint, M. (1954). Analytic training and training analysis. In: *Primary Love and Psycho-analytic Technique* (pp. 275–285). London: Tavistock, 1952 [reprinted 1965].

Balint, M. (1957). *The Doctor, his Patient and the Illness.* New York: International Universities Press.

Balint, M. (1959). *Thrills and Regressions.* New York: International Universities.

Balint, M. (1968). *The Basic Fault: Therapeutic Aspects of Regression.* London: Tavistock.

Balint, M., & Balint, E. (1961). *Psychotherapeutic Techniques in Medicine.* London: Tavistock.

Benjamin, W. (2002). *The Arcades Project* (Edited by R. Tiedemann). New York: Belknap Press.

Berger, J. (1967). *A Fortunate Man: The Story of a Country Doctor.* London: Allen Lane [reprinted London: Canongate, 2015].

Berlin, I. (1958). Two concepts of liberty. In: H. Hardy & R. Hausheer (Eds.), *The Proper Study of Mankind: An Anthology of Essays* (pp. 191–242). London: Pimlico, 1998.

Bernfeld, S. (1962). On psychoanalytic training. *Psychoanalytic Quarterly, 31*: 453–482.

Bleuler, E. (1911). *Dementia Praecox or the Group of Schizophrenias.* New York: International Universities, 1950.

Bollas, C. (2007). *The Freudian Moment.* London: Karnac.

Campkin, M. (1986). Is there a place for Balint in vocational training? *Journal of the Association of Course Organizers, 1*: 100–104.

Camus, A. (1942). *The Myth of Sisyphus*. London: Hamish Hamilton, 1955.

Carroll, L. (1865). Alice's Adventures in Wonderland. In: *The Annotated Alice: The Definitive Edition*. London: Penguin, 2000.

Cavafy, C. P. (1928). "In a large Greek colony, 200 BC". In: G. Savidis (Ed.), *Collected Poems*. London: Chatto & Windus, 1990.

Deutsch, F., & Murphy, W. F. (1955). *The Clinical Interview*. New York: International Universities.

Dispaux, M. -F. (2006). Candidates: obstacles in the process of supervision. Address at the EPF Forum on Education, Budapest, October 2005.

Dupont, J. (1988). Introduction. In: J. Dupont (Ed.), *The Clinical Diary of Sándor Ferenczi* (pp. xi–xxvii). Cambridge, MA: Harvard University Press.

Eliot, T. S. (1936). "Burnt Norton". In: *Collected Poems 1909–1935*. London: Faber & Faber [reprinted 1975].

Ferenczi, S. (1928). The elasticity of psychoanalytic technique. In: M. Balint (Ed.), *Final Contributions to the Problems and Methods of Psychoanalysis* (pp. 87–101). London: Hogarth, 1955.

Ferenczi, S. (1931). Child analysis in the analysis of adults. *International Journal of Psycho-analysis, 12*: 468–482.

Ferenczi, S. (1932). *The Clinical Diary of Sándor Ferenczi* (Ed. J. Dupont). Cambridge, MA: Harvard University Press, 1988.

Ferenczi, S. (1933). Confusion of tongues between adults and the child. In: M. Balint (Ed.), *Final Contributions to the Problems and Methods of Psycho-analysis* (pp. 156–167). London: Hogarth, 1955.

Forrester, J. (1990). *The Seductions of Psycho-analysis: Freud, Lacan and Derrida*. Cambridge: Cambridge University.

Freud, S. (1900a). *The Interpretation of Dreams*. S.E., 5: 588–609. London: Hogarth.

Freud, S. (1905a). On psychotherapy. *S.E., 7*: 255–268. London: Hogarth.

Freud, S. (1912e). Recommendations to physicians practising psycho-analysis. *S.E., 12*: 109–120. London: Hogarth.

Freud, S. (1912–1913). *Totem and Taboo*. S.E., 13: 1–162. London: Hogarth.

Freud, S. (1913c). On beginning the treatment (further recommendations on the technique of psycho-analysis I). *S.E., 12*: 121–144. London: Hogarth.

Freud, S. (1919a). Lines of advance in psycho-analytic therapy. *S.E., 17*: 157–168). London: Hogarth.

Freud, S. (1919e). "A child is being beaten": A contribution to the study of the origin of sexual perversions. *S.E., 17*: 175–204. London: Hogarth.

Freud, S. (1919j). On the teaching of psycho-analysis in universities. *S.E., 17*: 169–173. London: Hogarth.

Freud, S. (1923a). Two encyclopaedia articles. *S.E., 18*: 233–259. London: Hogarth.

Freud, S. (1926e). *The Question of Lay Analysis: Conversations with an Impartial Person. S.E., 20*: 177–258. London: Hogarth.

Freud, S. (1927c). *The Future of an Illusion. S.E., 21*: 1–56. London: Hogarth.

Freud, S. (1933a). Revision of the theory of dreams. *S.E., 22*: 7–30. London: Hogarth.

Freud, S. (1965a). *A Psycho-analytic Dialogue: The Letters of Sigmund Freud and Karl Abraham, 1907–1926*. London: Hogarth.

Freud, S., & Breuer, J. (1895d). *Studies on Hysteria. S.E., 2*: 185–251. London: Hogarth.

Freud, S., & Ferenczi, S. (2000). *The Correspondence of Sigmund Freud and Sándor Ferenczi (Volume 3: 1920–1933)* (E. Brabant, E. Falzeder & P. Giampeier-Deutsch (Eds.)). Cambridge, MA: Harvard University Press.

Green, A. (1986). *On Private Madness*. London: Hogarth.

Haynal, A. (1988). *The Technique at Issue: Controversies in Psychoanalysis from Freud and Ferenczi to Michael Balint*. London: Karnac.

Haynal, A. (2002). *Disappearing and Reviving: Sándor Ferenczi in the History of Psycho-analysis*. London: Karnac.

Heaney, S. (1996). "Mycenae Lookout". In: *The Spirit Level*. London: Faber & Faber.

Heimann, P. (1942). A contribution to the problem of sublimation and its relation to processes of internalization. In: M. Tonnesmann (Ed.), *About Children and Children-No-Longer* (pp. 26–45). London: Tavistock, 1989.

Heimann, P. (1949). Some notes on the psycho-analytic concept of introjected objects. In: M. Tonnesmann (Ed.), *About Children and Children-No-Longer* (pp. 61–72). London: Tavistock, 1989.

Heimann, P. (1952). A contribution to the re-evaluation of the Oedipus complex: the early stages. In: M. Tonnesmann (Ed.), *About Children and Children-No-Longer* (pp. 80–96). London: Tavistock, 1989.

Heimann, P. (1969). Postscript to "Dynamics of transference interpretations". In: M. Tonnesmann (Ed.), *About Children and Children-No-Longer* (pp. 252–261). London: Tavistock, 1989.

Jemstedt, A. (2008). The Sorrento experience: Chaos replaced by too much structure. In: D. Tuckett (Ed.), *Psychoanalysis Comparable and Incomparable: The Evolution of a Method to Describe and Compare Psychoanalytic Approaches*. London: Routledge.

Kahn, L. (2013). 26th conference of the European Psychoanalytic Federation 22 March 2013 La Limite et le passage. Unpublished.

Khan, M. M. R. (1969). On the clinical provision of frustrations, recognitions, and failures in the analytic situation: An essay on Dr. Michael Balint's researches on the theory of psychoanalytic technique. *International Journal of Psycho-analysis*, *50*: 237–248.

Khan, M. M. R. (1979). *Alienation in Perversions*. London: Hogarth.

King, P., & Steiner, R. (1991). *The Freud–Klein Controversies 1941–45*. London: Tavistock.

Kraepelin, E. (1887). Lectures in Clinical Psychiatry (facsimile of the 1904 edition). New York: Hafner, 1968.

Lacan, J. (1975). *The Seminar of Jacques Lacan: Book I, Freud's Papers on Technique 1953–1954*. Cambridge: Cambridge University Press, 1988.

Lacan, J. (1978). *The Seminar of Jacques Lacan: Book II, The Ego in Freud's Theory and in the Technique of Psycho-analysis 1954–1955*. London: Norton, 1988.

Laplanche, J., & Pontalis, J. -B. (1967). *The Language of Psycho-analysis*. London: Hogarth, 1973.

Laufer, M. (1976). The central masturbation fantasy, the final sexual organization, and adolescence. *The Psychoanalytic Study of the Child*, *31*: 297–316.

Leader, D. (2010). Some thoughts on supervision. *British Journal of Psychotherapy*, *26*: 228–241.

Mandela, N. (1964). Brief notes in the event of a death sentence. In: A. Sampson, *Mandela: The Authorised Biography*. London: Harper Collins, 1999.

Marty, P., & de M'Uzan, M. (1963). La pensée opératoire. *Revue française de psychanalyse*, *27*: 345–356.

Marx, K. (1867). *Capital: Critique of Political Economy: The Process of Capitalist Production*. London: Allen & Unwin, 1928 [reprinted 1946].

Moorhouse, P. (1996). *Leon Kossoff*. London: Tate Gallery.

Müller, W. (1824). "The Hurdy-Gurdy Man". In: I. Bostridge (Trans.), *Schubert's Winter Journey: Anatomy of an Obsession*. London: Faber & Faber, 2015.

Nunberg, H. (1959). Introduction. In: H. Nunberg & E. Federn (Eds.), *Minutes of the Vienna Psychoanalytic Society (Volume 1: 1906–1908)*. New York: International Universities, 1962.

Ogden, T. H. (1989). *The Primitive Edge of Experience*. Lanham, MD: Rowman & Littlefield.

Ogden, T. H. (1992). Comments on transference and countertransference in the initial analytic meeting. *Psychoanalytic Inquiry*, *12*: 225–247.

Parsons, M. (2014). *Living Psychoanalysis: From Theory to Experience*. Hove: Routledge.

Parsons, M. (2015). Faith in psychoanalysis. *Bulletin of the British Psychoanalytical Society*, *51*: 14–22.

Proust, M. (1921). *Sodom and Gomorrah*. London: Penguin, 2002.

Reich, W. (1933). *Character Analysis*. New York: Orgone Institute [reprinted 1949].

Rickman, J. (1951). Number and the human sciences. In: W. C. M. Scott (Ed.), *Selected Contributions to Psychoanalysis*. London: Hogarth, 1957.

Sidley, P. (2001). Drug companies sue South African government over generics. *British Medical Journal, 322*: 447.

Sklar, J. (2011). *Landscapes of the Dark: History, Trauma, Psychoanalysis*. London: Karnac.

Stewart, H. (1996). *Michael Balint: Object Relations Pure and Applied*. London: Routledge.

Terr, L. C. (1988). What happens to early memories of trauma? A study of twenty children under age five at the time of documented traumatic events. *Journal of the American Academy of Child and Adolescent Psychiatry, 27*: 96–104.

Tonnesmann, M. (1989). Editor's introduction. In: M. Tonnesmann (Ed.), *About Children and Children-No-Longer* (pp. 10–25). London: Tavistock.

Tuckett, D. (Ed.). (2008). *Psychoanalysis Comparable and Incomparable: The Evolution of a Method to Describe and Compare Psychoanalytic Approaches*. London: Routledge.

Tuckett, D. (2008). Reflection and evolution: Developing the two-step method. In: D. Tuckett (Ed.), *Psychoanalysis Comparable and Incomparable: The Evolution of a Method to Describe and Compare Psychoanalytic Approaches*. London: Routledge.

Wegner, P. (1992). The opening scene and the importance of the countertransference in the initial psychoanalytic interview. In: B. Reith, S. Lagerlöf, P. Crick, M. Møller, & E. Skale (Eds.), *Initiating Psychoanalysis: Perspectives* (pp. 225–242). London: Routledge, 2011.

Wegner, P. (2014). Process-orientated psychoanalytical work in initial interviews and the importance of the opening scene. *International Journal of Psycho-analysis, 95*: 511.

Winnicott, D. W. (1947). Hate in the countertransference. In: *Through Paediatrics to Psycho-analysis* (pp. 194–203). London: Hogarth, 1975.

Winnicott, D. W. (1951). Transitional objects and transitional phenomena: A study of the first *not-me* possession. *International Journal of Psycho-analysis, 34*: 89–97.

Winnicott, D. W. (1958). The capacity to be alone. *International Journal of Psycho-analysis, 39*: 416–420.

Winnicott, D. W. (1971). *Playing and Reality*. London: Tavistock [reprinted Harmondsworth: Pelican, 1974].

Woolf, V. (1937). Craftsmanship. In: *The Death of the Moth and Other Essays*. London: Hogarth, 1981.

Zetzel, E. R. (1968). The so-called good hysteric. *International Journal of Psycho-analysis, 49*: 256–260.

INDEX